Early Childhood Intervention

Early Childhood Intervention: Shaping the Future for Children with Special Needs and Their Families

Volume 1: Contemporary Policy and Practices Landscape

Volume 2: Proven and Promising Practices

Volume 3: Emerging Trends in Research and Practice

Early Childhood Intervention

Shaping the Future for Children with Special Needs and Their Families

Volume 1

Contemporary Policy and Practices Landscape

Steven Eidelman
Editor

Christina Groark, set editor

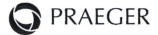 PRAEGER

AN IMPRINT OF ABC-CLIO, LLC
Santa Barbara, California • Denver, Colorado • Oxford, England

Northwest State Community College

Library of Congress Cataloging-in-Publication Data

Early childhood intervention : shaping the future for children with special needs and their
families / Christina Groark, set editor.
    p. cm.
  Includes bibliographical references and index.
    ISBN 978–0–313–37793–8 (hard copy : alk. paper) — ISBN 978–0–313–37794–5 (ebook)
    1. Children with disabilities–Education (Preschool)—United States. 2. Children with
disabilities—Services for—United States. 3. Child development–United States. 4. Child
welfare–United States. I. Groark, Christina J.
LC4019.2.E25   2011
371.9–dc22   2011011997

ISBN: 978–0–313–37793–8
EISBN: 978–0–313–37794–5

15 14 13 12 11   1 2 3 4 5

This book is also available on the World Wide Web as an eBook.
Visit www.abc-clio.com for details.

Praeger
An Imprint of ABC-CLIO, LLC

ABC-CLIO, LLC
130 Cremona Drive, P.O. Box 1911
Santa Barbara, California 93116-1911

This book is printed on acid-free paper ∞

Manufactured in the United States of America

For Paul, my son, and all children with special needs who deserve the best start in life that society in general, policy makers, professionals, and families can give them, and to those who advocate for them, thank you.

Contents

Preface and Acknowledgments

This series of three volumes is about special services known as *early intervention* or *early childhood special education* (EI/ECSE) provided to young children with special needs and their families. As the terms imply, these services provide support early in a child's life, even as early as birth, until the age of school entry. Specifically, early intervention as found in Part C of the IDEA 2004 Statute (P.L. 108-446) is defined as health, educational, and/or therapeutic services that are provided under public supervision and are designed to meet the developmental needs of an infant or toddler who has a developmental delay or a disability. At the discretion of each state, services can also be provided to children who are considered to be *at risk* of developing substantial delays if services are not provided. These services must be provided by qualified personnel and, to the maximum extent appropriate, must be provided in natural environments including the home and community settings in which children without disabilities participate. Early childhood special education (ECSE), as found in Part B, Section 619 of the IDEA, intends for smooth transition of a child from EI to ECSE. It stipulates that the local education agency will participate in the transition planning of a child from early intervention (Part C) to early childhood special education for a preschool-aged child the year she turns 3 years of age. The child may receive all the early intervention services listed on her service plan until her third birthday. Then she must be assessed as eligible for ECSE services

Why is this field important? First, it is scientifically known that early childhood is a time of significant brain development and substantial growth in every domain of all children's development. Second, it is widely accepted that at this time, all learning takes place in the context of relationships, and that families are central to these relationships. Therefore, for better child outcomes, short and long term, families must be involved at all levels. Third, professionals serving eligible children and families must be on the same page with the families, the children, and each other by coordinating their work and being focused on the skills that are important in the individual child's life. Fourth, this field is important because it demonstrates a connection between instruction and developmental outcomes that benefit children with or without disabilities. For example, the design of certain curricula, individualized educational programs, universal design for environments, tiered teaching methods, and other practices in these volumes are good strategies for all children, not only those with special needs.

But why attend to this particular population of children and families here and now? The prevalence of children with special needs worldwide as well as nationally is increasing. In 1991–1992, the prevalence of children with disabilities in the United States was estimated at 5.75 percent (http://www.cdc.gov/mmwr/PDF/wk/mm4433.pdf). In a more recent review (*Pediatrics* [2008], *121*, e1503–e1509) by Rosenberg, Zhang, and Robinson, the prevalence of developmental delays of children born in the United States in 2001 and eligible for Part C early intervention was indicated at 13 percent.

This growing prevalence also points to economic and public health concerns. Developmental delay, when attended to appropriately earlier in life, is shown to be lessened and thereby alleviate costs to the public. Typically, the estimated lifetime cost for those born in 2000 with a developmental disability is expected to total (based on 2003 dollars) $51.2 billion for people with intellectual disabilities, $11.5 billion for people with cerebral palsy, $2.1 billion for people who are deaf or have hearing loss, and $2.5 billion for people with vision impairment (http://www.cdc.gov/ncbddd/dd/ddsurv.htm). Early services work to significantly reduce these costs.

Also, as society, the economy, and all aspects of life are becoming more globally interdependent, it is our responsibility to help all children reach their potentials and contribute positively to our future. Our society needs a trained, talented, and diverse workforce. We cannot afford to lose the potential of such an important and large sector of children.

In addition to growing prevalence and the need for a diverse workforce, special needs affect all types of families. There is no culture, ethnic group, gender, geographic area, or socioeconomic status group that does not include children with special needs. Special needs and disabilities are inordinately diverse in terms of diagnosis, variability within a diagnosis, intensity, spectrum of characteristics, age of impact, multiplicity, and combinations of disabilities. Further, all children, typically developing or not, need some individualized attention, instruction, and care. They are not little adults. They learn by different styles and at different rates.

Because of this diversity and the importance of the development of this cohort of children, the editors worked diligently to be sure that the most current and best available research is combined with professional experiences, wisdom, and values; clinical expertise; and family-child perspectives. Although no rock was left unturned in the selection of topics and contributors, there was some difficulty in selecting topics. The advisors, editors, and publishers felt strongly that this series is to be of utility to a variety of professionals, parents, practitioners, policy makers, service trainers, students, academics, and scholars, including those not directly related to this field (e.g., a lawyer who is interested in policy, a parent who wants to know about the best supports for her child). Although we strongly intended to have the three volumes provide breadth to the readers, we still wanted them to be as comprehensive as possible. Once the topics were agreed upon, authors were easy to select because we invited the best in the field who could communicate the issues in an accurate, precise, and understandable way. Therefore, information was gathered from experience and scientific evidence by the best in the fields of early intervention and early childhood special education policy and law, medicine and health sciences, and education and child welfare, among others.

So the reader will find that the scope of this series is broad but still covers the critical components of early intervention and early childhood special education. It is organized into three volumes in such a way that readers can skim through each to find the areas of particular interest to them. The chapters within the three volumes are intended to answer key questions regarding how this field works. For instance, how do we identify children needing early intervention or early childhood special education and recognize them as early as possible? Where does this detection and subsequent service take place? Who works in early intervention, and what is their training? What is the families' role in all of this, and what are their rights? How does that role differ in early intervention compared to early childhood special education? Which programs, or what parts of programs, work best, and for whom? What does it cost to provide this service, and how effective is it? What are still some of the unknowns of this field (which is relatively young compared to other fields of study)?

Specifically, Volume 1, *Contemporary Policy and Practices Landscape*, begins with a historical perspective of this field. It then relates state policies and various attempts to implement them and international laws and sample country responses to the care, education, and development of children with disabilities. This volume also considers who provides these services; their training, background, and experiences; and evaluation of programs for quality and cost-effectiveness. Policies regarding children with special needs nationally and internationally tell us the rights of children and families. Sometimes they even tell us what should be provided and when. However, they do not tell us *how* to implement quality programs; thus, the need for Volume 2.

You will see, therefore, that the chapters in Volume 2, *Proven and Promising Practices in Early Intervention/Early Childhood Special Education*, cover the best available practices that are currently used and studied throughout the field of early intervention. These chapters include information on programs such as Early Head Start and Head Start and new, exciting model strategies and techniques in intervening with children with challenging behaviors, mental health diagnoses, sensory processing, and others. We were fortunate to find the best professionals in the fields of early intervention and early childhood special education, including individuals from occupational therapy, speech and language pathology, psychology, policy development, technology use with children, early literacy and math, teacher education, English-language learning, and specialists in visual and hearing impairments. Yet there is always room for new knowledge and improvement. That is what we hope we captured in Volume 3.

Volume 3, *Emerging Trends in Research and Practice*, creatively takes the reader into the realm of possibilities. It helps the reader think about needs of expanding or emerging populations such as culturally and linguistically diverse families and the need for schools to be prepared for learners with a wide range of needs and abilities. This volume also invites reflection on issues that are not totally resolved, like crossing systems in the delivery of services, how do we get over the financial and administrative silos in these public systems, and how do we get professionals and bureaucrats to work together to cross these systems? However, this volume also provides solutions to current issues that should be considered, advocated for, or debated, such as the Recognition and Response tiered model of instruction.

Finally, the chapters in Volume 3 point us in the direction of future research and trials of models and strategies. For instance, we need to make the best use of technology and research-based practices. Another example includes child progress monitoring and accountability. Monitoring and accountability have evolved over the years, and better practices actually may include simpler procedures. But are we capturing the complexities of teaching and learning? Do we really understand the needs of children with special needs and how to best engage their families and integrate a variety of professional recommendations for the most effective program? Finding these answers will demand a lot from professionals (e.g., to follow professional practices such as DEC-NAEYC), from researchers (e.g., to develop and test evidenced based practices), and from the public in general (e.g., to advocate).

All three volumes contain special features like matrices, graphs, and diagrams to stimulate readers not only in what is, but in what could be. They are different from other works in that they provide the state of the art in the field while considering the antecedents and the future prospective in the field. They are intended to be appealing to anyone interested in children, especially children with special needs, and to provide enough information to continue and grow that interest.

* * *

I would like to thank many people for their contributions to the creation, writing, editing, and production of this series. First, the volume editors, Steven Eidelman, Susan P. Maude, and Louise A. Kaczmarek, all of whom are first-rate professionals, child advocates, and early interventionists whom I relied upon heavily for chapter ideas, finding the best authors in the field, volume editing, writing chapters for the volumes, and fabulous contributions to the entire enterprise. There would be no series without them.

Second, my assistants, Mary Ellen Colella, Amy Gee, Mary Louise Kaminski, and Kaitlin Moore, who kept me organized, edited me and reedited me, and checked details when I could no longer see the trees through the forest.

In addition, thank you to our illustrious advisers. They came from so many different professions with the highest level of understanding of the nature of the children in these services and of what is needed by our readers. I appreciate their willingness to share their expertise openly and candidly.

And to my students, Amber Harris-Fillius, Claudia Ovalle-Ramirez, Robin Sweitzer, and Wen Chi Wang, thank you for their thorough reviews of the chapters. I learned a lot from them.

Finally, thank you to my family: Brian, Patti, Stephanie, and Paul, for teaching me about children and families and for their patience and encouragement throughout this work.

Chapter 1

Historical Perspectives

Barbara J. Smith and Beth Rous

Volumes have been written on the theoretical, scientific, social, and policy foundations of early childhood intervention (see for example, Shonkoff & Meisels, 2003). This introductory chapter attempts to provide a summary perspective on that rich history.

There are two key terms related to early childhood intervention used in this chapter: early intervention and early childhood special education. In *Early Childhood Education: An International Encyclopedia*, edited by New and Cochran (2007), these terms are described. Smith and Guralnick (2007) describe early intervention as the body of "policies, systems, programs, services, and supports provided to vulnerable young children and/or their families to maximize a child's development" (pp. 329–330). Further, Smith and Guralnick point out that "the concept of early intervention implies that: (1) acting earlier rather than later results in important effects not gained if action is delayed, and (2) action is needed beyond that typically available and is based on specific circumstances and unique child and family characteristics" (p. 330).

Early childhood special education (ECSE) is described by Mallory (2007) as "a field characterized by grounded theory, practices, and applied research concerned with the causes and consequences of disability in the first eight years of life. The field has evolved since its inception in the 1960s and 1970s based on increasingly more sophisticated understandings of the nature of early childhood disability" (p. 321).

As used in this chapter, early intervention can be viewed as a term encompassing the array of services and policies established for improving the developmental trajectory of young children, from birth to age eight, with special needs and their families. Early childhood special education (ECSE) is the profession that establishes the parameters for professional standards, program standards, and approaches, and embodies the theoretical and scientific foundations for the field.

This chapter provides the theoretical and scientific history as well as the sociopolitical roots of ECSE and early intervention.

THEORETICAL FOUNDATIONS

Mallory (2007) describes ECSE as having evolved from the fields of early childhood education (ECE) and special education, but that it is "more than the sum of these two components; it now represents a distinct body of professional knowledge, practice, and policy" (p. 321).

EARLY CHILDHOOD EDUCATION FOUNDATIONS

ECSE and early intervention are grounded in key theoretical foundations of ECE. One such foundational theory is early childhood as a distinct period of human development characterized by approaches to learning and interpreting the world differently from those of adults. Second, ECSE and early intervention embody the ECE notion that development is sequential but responsive to environmental factors that affect that sequence or trajectory. Twentieth-century writers and theorists shifted the concept of human development as a fixed sequence of stages to the concept that a child's development is affected not only by nature, or the characteristics of the child at birth, but also by nurture, or those things the environment provides. This view of young children was directly influenced by human ecologists. This perspective views human development as an interaction between the growing human being and the contexts or environment with which it interacts (Cochran, 2007). As we will describe later in this chapter and in greater detail in Chapter 2, many of the key issues and practices in the field of ECSE and early intervention today reflect this concept of the importance of the child's interaction with its environment, such as inclusion (e.g., children and families having access to services and community opportunities).

Early education movements in the early 1800s emphasized these theories as well as the role early education could play in ensuring an educated citizenry and transforming society (Bauer, Johnson, Ulrich, Denno, & Carr, 1998). In the United States, the first systematic developments in ECE were the establishment of kindergartens with the goal of supporting social and emotional readiness for formal schooling. In 1873, Susan Blow founded the first public kindergarten in St. Louis and by 1883, every public school in St. Louis had a kindergarten class-room. Day nurseries were established in the mid-1800s with the goal of providing young children of working parents with custodial care in home-like settings. With changing values related to women working out of the home, and particularly with the women's suffrage move-ment in the early 1900s, other forms of ECE developed. Nursery schools were established in the early 1900s primarily by and for middle-class families and focused more on education and social emotional development of young children and to serve as informa-tional resources for parents. As theories of the developing child and the developing brain were advancing, so too did efforts emerge to show effective ways of teaching young children. In the 1920s, the National Association of Nursery School Educators (NANE) was founded. In 1927, the National Committee on Nursery Schools recommended a four-year college degree for nursery school teachers (Darragh, 2010).

In the 1930s and 1940s, the Great Depression created high unem-ployment, and World War II created the need for women to work out-side the home to fill both jobs left by men who were in the military and jobs created to support the war effort. Therefore, caring for chil-dren outside of the home became a necessity. The Works Progress Administration in 1933 supported nursery schools so that out-of-work teachers could have jobs. In the 1940s, the federal government pro-vided funding for child care so that women could work in war-related industries (Bauer et al., 1998). Views about ECE and the availability of ECE settings continued to evolve with the women's equity movement. The Equal Pay Act of 1963 and Titles VII and IX of the Civil Rights Act of 1964 ushered in federal equal rights for women and girls in educa-tion and employment as well as a growth in child care opportunities (Darragh, 2010).

These historic events expanded early education as a system and as a profession. However, during this period, young children with disabil-ities received little attention.

SPECIAL EDUCATION FOUNDATIONS

The second theoretical foundation of ECSE and early intervention according to Mallory (2007) is the field of special education. At roughly the same time period in the nineteenth century that theories associated with early childhood as a distinct period of human development with its own learning characteristics emerged, so too emerged an interest in atypical human development. This interest and documentation of developmental disabilities and mental illness led to a subsequent movement to address the needs of these populations. Early approaches to address or "treat" disability were to create institutions to house individuals away from society.

The eighteenth and nineteenth centuries brought theories advancing the idea that young children's development is not predetermined but is influenced by environmental factors. This same notion was put forward regarding the developmental trajectory of people with disabilities. Seguin and Itard proposed that children with disabilities could learn and were not possessed by demons or need to be incarcerated (Bauer et al., 1998). Inspired by this work and Seguin's move to the United States from France, educational programs for people with mental retardation expanded, albeit in residential institutions, and by the end of the nineteenth century these institutions were well established and committed to education and to some degree the eventual inclusion into the community of persons with disabilities (Shonkoff & Meisels, 2003).

However, in the early twentieth century, influenced by those who supported the eugenics movement, the residential institutions were refocused from training and possible social integration to custodial care. This movement justified racist and immigration restrictions and compulsory sterilization (Shonkoff & Meisels, 2003). Work on the new Binet Intelligence Test involved administering the test to newly arriving immigrants at Ellis Island to identify the "feebleminded progeny of the foreign hordes" (Gilhool, 1995, p. 13, in Bauer et al., 1998), and states supported public institutions to separate individuals with disabilities because they were considered dangerous. Some states went so far as to make it a criminal offense for parents to refuse institutionalization (Gilhool, 1995). Thus, according to Shonkoff and Meisels (2003), "The psychology community's harsh rhetoric challenged the early optimism of special education and residential institutions were transformed into dreary warehouses for neglected and forgotten individuals" (p. 9).

With the expansion of public schooling in the United States at the turn of the twentieth century, the field of special education reemerged with a focus on diagnosis, and an acceptance that learning and development are not fixed but rather can be affected by the environment including education. Over the next four decades, testing of recruits for World Wars I and II revealed many people were living typical lives with disabilities, and with the return of the veterans with war-related disabilities, the view of disability began to change, resulting in a growing recognition of a need to provide support and services (Bauer et al., 1998).

In the mid-1960s, findings from researchers such as Skeels, Skeels and Dye, and Kirk indicated that with enriched early experiences, the learning trajectories of young children with disabilities could be dramatically altered for the better (Bauer et al., 1998; Shonkoff & Meisels, 2003). At the same time, other educational theorists and researchers were looking at the relationship of children's characteristics and the quality of the environment. Benjamin Bloom (1964) and J. McVicker Hunt (1961) argued that intelligence is not fixed, develops early, and is affected by early experiences. In the 1960s, this scientific and theoretical foundation along with strong support from the Kennedy administration led to states enacting legislation and social values changing resulting in expanded educational programs for children with disabilities. However, special education and early intervention services were largely confined to volunteer efforts and provided to children with disabilities in settings separate from their typically developing peers.

Caldwell (1973) described these various eras in special education as three distinct historical periods: (1) "forget and hide," (2) "screen and segregate," and (3) "identify and help." Allen and Schwartz (1996, p. 4) suggest that the current era could be captioned as "include and support" as described in Chapter 2.

SOCIOPOLITICAL FOUNDATIONS

As noted above, concurrent with the theoretical and scientific advances in the mid-1960s, public policy began to play a key role in the expansion of services and the development of systems for special education, early childhood education, ECSE, and early intervention. While research findings were establishing the importance of education in the lives of young children and those with disabilities, services were voluntary and not part of the mainstream education systems. Advocates began to turn to policy makers in an effort to establish more and better services for young children with special needs. States began to enact policies providing education for school-age children with disabilities, special education as a profession grew, the Kennedy administration provided strong support for services for people with disabilities, the federal Bureau of the Education of the Handicapped (BEH) within the Department of Health, Education, and Welfare was established, and federal support for research and development and personnel preparation in special education was provided. Additionally, an increase in concern and advocacy over marginalized populations and a call for equal protection of the law and fairness in society resulted in monumental advances for young children with disabilities, and other special needs such as living in poverty.

LEVELS AND BRANCHES OF GOVERNMENT AND POLICY

ECSE and early intervention have essential roots in public policy. To fully grasp this policy foundation, it is important to understand the structure of public policy and government in the United States. The U.S. Constitution outlines the governance of the United States. This structure is comprised of levels of government as outlined in the Constitution—federal and state levels. Each of these levels has its own governance that creates policy. At each level, there are three branches of government—legislative, executive, and judicial—all of which are designed to limit and balance power.

First and foremost to understanding past and present sociopolitical issues in ECSE and early intervention, is the delineation between the two levels of government: federal and state. The limitation of power was key to the writing of the U.S. Constitution—limitation of power of government over the individual, and limitation of the power of the federal government over state governments. The 10th Amendment of the Constitution was added to clarify that the powers not delegated in the Constitution to the federal government "are reserved to States respectively, or to the people." This form of government, federal and several sovereign states, is referred to as "federalism." As described below, ECSE and early intervention policy has been developed at both the federal and state levels. It is important to note there is a tension or balance between the federal and state governments as to the appropriate role of each in education and human services. The concept of "federalism" is important to understanding this balance and the conversation between policy makers at the different levels of government. A good example of this tension is the attempt of the Reagan administration in the early 1980s to repeal the Education for All Handicapped Children Act, under the argument that such education matters belonged to the states and not the federal government. Advocates and supporters worked to convince the administration of the need for a federal presence in establishing a right to an education for children with disabilities and persuaded the administration to with-draw its proposal.

As described above, the U.S. governance structure at both the federal and state levels is comprised of three branches that serve as checks and balances on the power of each. As described in the Constitution, the branches are legislative (which passes laws), executive (which imple-ments the laws), and judicial (which interprets the laws). Article I of the Constitution describes the legislative powers at the federal level as resting with the Congress. At the state level, the legislative branch is the state legislature. Article II describes the executive branch at the federal level as the president, which includes the president's cabinet and agencies such as the Department of Education or Department of Health and Human Services. At the state level, the executive branch is the governor, state cabinet and agencies such as the state departments of education, health, or human services. Article III describes the third branch of government as the judicial branch, which at the federal level is the Supreme Court and federal district court system. At the state level, the judicial branch is the state court system including the state Supreme Court.

As noted above, there is a tension about what type of policy should rest with what level (federal or state). Policy makers and advocates debate the appropriate role of federal and state governments in areas such as whether the federal government should intervene in states' delivery of services (see the legal history of services to children with disabilities described later in this chapter) or whether the more appro-priate role of federal policy is to entice or provide incentives to states to meet certain goals versus mandating them. These enticements or incentives may be voluntary grants to begin services to children, or grants to agencies or programs to research and disseminate best prac-tices that may eventually lead to widespread use of such services and approaches. As described below, advocates argued that the federal government needed to establish a right to an education for children with disabilities because states had failed to do so even with incen-tives, and because the federal government could provide requirements that would cross state lines thus ensuring some continuity of services to children and families regardless of the state in which they resided. Throughout the following section, there are examples of the federal role in providing: (1) resources and direction for non-mandatory serv-ices, which we will refer to as incentives and policies directed at improving the quality of services; and (2) mandating services, which we will refer to as ensuring access to services. Also, below are examples of how the various branches of government have been used to advance services to children with disabilities.

THE ROLE OF POLICY IN ECSE AND EARLY INTERVENTION

Public policy has played two major roles in ECSE and early intervention: (1) encouraging states and localities to provide services and providing resources and guidance about best practice; and (2) requiring states to provide services and to establish systems for doing so. By the mid-1960s, the research on the effects of early experience and child development led to two major federal initiatives that paved the way to where we are today in ECSE and early intervention. These two policy initiatives represent the federal government providing incentives and guidance to states to provide services versus requiring them to do so. The first, Project Head Start, a federal program of early education and other supportive services for young children living in poverty, was enacted in 1964 under the Economic Opportunity Act as a component of the "War on Poverty" of the Johnson administration. Head Start was established to provide early intervention for young children at risk for school failure due to poverty. In 1972, Head Start programs were required to allocate 10 percent of its enrollment for children with disabilities. This requirement not only resulted in the first national early intervention services for young children with disabilities, but also made a national statement about the importance of serving young children with disabilities with their typically developing peers rather than separately.

The second major policy milestone during this period was the Handicapped Children's Early Education Program (HCEEP) enacted by Congress in 1968 to develop research and demonstration projects aimed at discovering new and better approaches to working with young children with disabilities. DeWeerd (1977) and Hebbeler, Smith, and Black (1991) described the contribution the HCEEP program had in developing a body of knowledge and effective models and interventions. DeWeerd noted that by 1968, Congress recognized one reason there were so few services for young children with disabilities was the shortage of models of programs that were effective. Thus they established HCEEP to provide grants to:

1. Support research on effective practices
2. Provide grants to universities for student stipends to encourage students to study and become ECSE providers

3. Develop, demonstrate, and outreach information on effective models of ECSE
4. Develop a national center to provide technical assistance to programs and states on how to deliver ECSE

The body of research, demonstration programs, scientific literature, and a national network of advocates that resulted from the HCEEP program led to: (1) widespread awareness of the positive effects early intervention could have on young children's development and future; (2) advocacy groups that included family members, scientists, and program personnel; and (3) ECSE teacher degree programs established at the university level across the nation.

A major unintended result of this comprehensive initiative was the establishment of the professional association, the Division for Early Childhood (DEC) of the Council for Exceptional Children (CEC). DEC established the first research journal, the *Journal of Early Intervention*, and an annual professional conference, and it provided a platform for advancing professional standards, programs standards, and public policies that promote best practices for optimizing the developmental outcomes of young children with special needs, including children with disabilities, children at risk for disabilities, and children living in poverty.

While HCEEP was helping to develop the field of early intervention and ECSE, other important sociopolitical events were happening. By the mid-1970s it was estimated that one million school-age children with disabilities were not receiving an education (Weintraub & Abeson, 1976). Building on the right to education precedent set in the 1954 *Brown v. Board of Education* court ruling, which established a right to equal education for all children regardless of race, the 1970s saw several court cases and other policies advance the right to education for children with disabilities. In 1971, the landmark *Pennsylvania Association for Retarded Children v. Commonwealth of Pennsylvania* lawsuit established the right to an education for all school-age children with mental retardation. In 1972, in *Mills v. Board of Education*, the court in the District of Columbia established a right to an education for all children with disabilities of school age. These court cases found that under the equal protection clause of the 14th Amendment to the U.S. Constitution that if education is provided by the state to one group, it must be provided to all. The interpretation of the equal protection clause was evolving from ensuring equal access to the same resources, to "equal access to differing resources for equal objectives" (Weintraub &

Abeson, 1976, p. 8). Soon, state legislatures and other court cases followed, and children with disabilities were winning the right to an education, to due process during important decisions such as assessment, to diagnosis and placement in special education, and to have services provided in the "least restrictive environment." This right to education movement culminated in 1975 with the Education for All Handicapped Children Act (P.L. 94-142), which was created by amendment to the Education of the Handicapped Act (later named the Individuals with Disabilities Education Act, or IDEA). This new law mandated states to provide a free, appropriate public education to all school-age children with disabilities in the least restrictive environment and according to a written Individualized Education Program (IEP). P.L. 94-142, while not requiring states to serve very young children, provided financial incentives to states to provide preschool education to children with disabilities younger than age six.

In 1984, based upon research findings on the efficacy of early intervention services and the social value of supporting families and children, Congress established a new program under HCEEP that provided federal funds to states for planning, developing, and implementing statewide services for children with disabilities from birth to five years of age. Again, this was not a mandate, but an incentive program. In 1984, about half the states had public policies for providing early intervention and education services to some portion of the population of young children with disabilities, ages 3–5, with 10 states providing some services from birth (Smith, 1988).

Building on these state efforts, and based on an accumulation of the federally funded efficacy research and development of effective practices and services under HCEEP, Congress passed P.L. 99-457 in 1986, the Education of the Handicapped Act Amendments of 1986. These amendments created what is now known as IDEA, Part C for infants and toddlers with disabilities and IDEA, Part B, Section 619 for preschool-aged children with disabilities. This law required states to lower the age from six to three for a free appropriate public education to children with disabilities under Part B. It also established a voluntary early intervention program of services for children with disabilities or at risk for disabilities from birth through age two under Part C. One of the architects of P.L. 99-457, Robert Silverstein, a congressional staff person involved in the writing of the law, gave a speech in 1988 (Silverstein, 1988) in which he quoted from materials sent to the Congress from the U.S. Department of Education in 1985 about the findings from the HCEEP program. The materials said: "Studies of the effectiveness of preschool education for the handicapped have demonstrated beyond doubt the economic and educational benefits of programs for young handicapped children. In addition the studies have shown the earlier intervention is started, the greater is the ultimate dollar savings and the higher is the rate of educational attainment by these handicapped children." Silverstein went on to say that information from states at that time indicated the number of preschool children with disabilities being served had leveled off over the years and the current incentives were not sufficient for all children to receive services, . . . "Some members of Congress thought that it was time to take advantage of 17 or so years of research showing the effectiveness of early intervention and mandate the provision of services for the birth to five population" (p. 10). Thus it is clear that a policy mandating states to provide services to young children with disabilities was built upon policies that provided incentives to states and policies that supported research and development of effective practices funded under the HCEEP program under EHA. However, it is also evident that the research funding and state incentives were not adequate, and that a policy requiring services was also needed if all children were to be served.

The effect of these policies is clear. State policies for providing services to young children with disabilities increased dramatically over the next decade. Smith and McKenna (1994) described the dramatic increase in state early intervention and preschool services between 1986 and 1992:

> In 1986, only 25 states had legal mandates for services to children under the age of 6. By 1992, however, all states had established policies that ensured that all eligible children had access to early intervention services from birth . . . in 1986 states were reportedly serving fewer than 30,000 infants as compared to nearly 250,000 by 1991. (p. 257)

In the 1980s and 1990s, there have been amendments to IDEA refining some of the early childhood provisions, but by and large, there have been few major federal initiatives in the early intervention arena. However, Early Head Start was established for birth-to-2-year-olds and contains the same 10 percent enrollment of children with disabilities requirements as the 3- to 5-year-old program. Funding for IDEA and Head Start has increased but is still not sufficient to appropriately serve all eligible children. A major milestone was the passage of the Americans with Disabilities Act (ADA) in 1990. While this is not early childhood legislation, it bans discrimination in public services such as child care and other early childhood settings. Therefore, children with disabilities gained the right to entry to many natural settings and environments through the ADA.

ISSUES AND TRENDS

Unfortunately, an unexpected turn of events occurred in the mid-1990s that affected the available resources at the federal level that were used to promote quality ECSE and early intervention services. A movement to reduce the size of the federal government led to the repeal of several programs, one of which was HCEEP. Therefore, there is currently no federal program solely dedicated to funding early intervention and ECSE research and development efforts. Research has traditionally been seen as an appropriate role of the federal government as it benefits all states and therefore should not be the burden of any one state. There are opportunities for research funding through other programs, but not at the level of the targeted HCEEP program. This development challenges states to establish the policies and structures to promote high-quality ECSE and early intervention services and systems. While most states will not significantly support research, there are other quality-enhancing policies and systems more likely to be implemented by states.

One approach to enhancing quality in states is the establishment of training, professional development, and technical assistance programs to support the use of effective practice at the local level. However, currently many states do not provide such supportive systems. Often, states provide support for short-term training sessions on particular topics of interest or concern. However, a growing body of research suggests training alone, without on-site coaching to provide opportunities for application of new strategies with feedback, does not result in a change of current practice by service providers. To achieve adoption of effective practice and strategies, providers need to receive information on the new practice, be provided with an opportunity to apply that practice, and receive supportive feedback (Blase, 2009; Fixsen, Naoom, Blase, Freidman, & Wallace, 2005; Joyce & Showers, 2002). To achieve this type of professional development and technical assistance system, states will need to develop policies and resources that may currently not be in place within the state. Further, while this is indicated as the most effective way to achieve high-quality services and systems, it will require a paradigm shift for states to establish and support such intensive technical assistance and training systems for early childhood programs. Blase (2009) described how states can approach building such a system, from designing basic technical assistance to programs that capitalize on their current readiness for coaching and other professional development approaches, to intensive technical assistance targeted at programs and systems. However, this approach can require a full systems-change effort, including resources, systems, and quality assurance mechanisms such as certification and licensing related to the evidence-based practices as well as data collection and evaluation systems tied to quality improvement efforts.

In addition to the theoretical, scientific, and policy foundations to early intervention and ECSE, by the 1990s there was also a social value that providing effective services and supports to young children with special needs and their families should be conducted in settings that are normal and include typically developing peers (Sandall, Hemmeter, Smith, & McLean, 2005). This concept of "inclusion" has been a focal point of early intervention and ECSE for the past 20 years. It has major ramifications of the field on policies, on personnel preparation, and on systems at the local, state, and federal levels. One of the major implications of the inclusion movement has been to bring the fields of ECSE and ECE together, not as one field but as two coordinated fields of knowledge necessary to meet the needs of all children (Smith & Bredekamp, 1998). While ECSE emanated partly from ECE, it diverged in many ways, not the least of which is in the development of different pedagogical approaches to teaching young children. Research has shown that young children with disabilities often need more structured, adult-directed teaching strategies to learn the same objectives as their typically developing peers (Smith, Miller, & Bredekamp, 1998). They may need adaptations to approaches, materials, and equipment, and they may need help in accessing the same curriculum as their peers. The two professional associations, the Division for Early Childhood (DEC) of the Council for Exceptional Children and the National Association for the Education of Young Children (NAEYC), have worked together since the early 1990s to establish a shared vision of inclusion, and to promulgate personnel and program recommendations for how to teach all children together. In 1993, DEC and NAEYC issued a position statement about the importance of inclusion. Subsequently they worked together to help early educators to blend the approaches and to see the teaching strategies as a continuum of effective strategies depending on the needs of the child. Rous describes

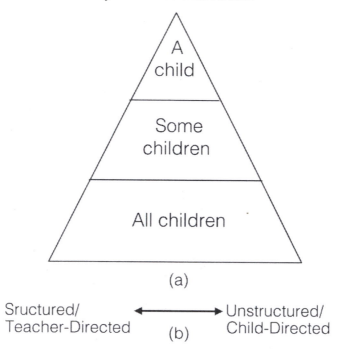

(a)

Sructured/   Unstructured/
Teacher-Directed   (b)   Child-Directed

**Figure 1.1   Conceptual models of individual appropriateness:
(a) Pyramid model. (b) Continuum model.**

in Chapter 2 how this early position on inclusion has been revised and
built upon by the two organizations.

Smith and Bredekamp in 1998, representing the two professional
associations, described the importance of early educators and early
childhood special educators collaborating in inclusive settings to bring
the full range of teaching approaches necessary for all children. They
described two conceptual models for viewing the ECE and ECSE
teaching practices: one as a pyramid, and one as a continuum, both
representing the range of strategies from those for all children to those
specialized strategies that some children may need some of the time
(see Figure 1.1).

In addition to conceptualizing shared teaching approaches and collaboration of personnel to effectively teach all children in an inclusive
environment, inclusion has also presented paradigm shifts in teacher
education, service system coordination, and accountability. Chapter 2
describes these issues in more detail.

While there have been many advances for young children with disabilities and their families, there remain many challenges. Young

children with disabilities have gained access to programs and services, but the quality and effectiveness of those services are still not funded and supported at a level suitable to promote the optimal development of all children. Other challenges include services in inclusive and natural environments (such as the family home or child care centers), family centeredness, transition from one system to another, and professional competence. While the federal role in ECSE policy has been and will likely continue to be primarily providing access to services, the role of states should be focused on the assurance that those services are of the highest quality necessary to ensure optimal developmental outcomes. This means states need to invest in training and technical assistance to programs to ensure that personnel have the skills they need to provide effective services. States need to link accountability measures to supports to programs in an effort to establish continuous improvement based upon those measures. States and universities need to establish personnel licensing standards that meet national recommendations from DEC and NAEYC.

Harkening back to the beginnings of the field of ECSE and early intervention services, it is imperative that advocates express to policy makers the importance of the relationship of the young child's development and the ecology of that child: the quality of that ecology (the knowledge and resources of the family, the health and educational services provided to the child and family, the accessibility and level that the community welcomes children with special needs, and professional competence) will determine the development of the child. Therefore, not only is early intervention the right thing to do, but it is imperative that it is done effectively.

In Chapter 2, we describe in more detail current programs and challenges in the field, particularly those related to the quality and inclusiveness of the early intervention and ECSE services provided to young children and their families across multiple service systems.

REFERENCES

Allen, K. E., & Schwartz, I. S. (1996). *The exceptional child: Inclusion in early childhood education.* Albany, NY: Delmar.

Bauer, A. M., Johnson, L. J., Ulrich, M., Denno, D. M., & Carr, V. W. (1998). A history of working with and for children. In L. Johnson, M. LaMontagne, P. Elgas, & A. Bauer (Eds.), *Early childhood education: Blending theory, blending practice.* Baltimore: Paul H. Brookes.

Blase, K. A. (2009). *Technical assistance to promote service and system change: Roadmap to effective intervention practices.* Technical Assistance Center on Social Emotional Intervention. Retrieved from http://www.challengingbehavior.org.

Bloom, B. S. (1964). *Stability and change in human characteristics.* New York: Wiley.

Caldwell, B. M. (1973). The importance of beginning early. In M. B. Karnes (Ed.), *Not all little wagons are red: The exceptional child's early years.* Arlington, VA: Council for Exceptional Children.

Cochran, M. (2007). Ecology of human development. In R. New & M. Cochran (Eds.), *Early childhood education: An international encyclopedia.* Westport, CT: Praeger.

Darragh, J. C. (2010). *Introduction to early childhood education.* Upper Saddle River, NJ: Pearson.

DeWeerd, J. (1977). Introduction. In J. Jordan, A. Hayden, M. Karnes, & M. Wood (Eds.), *Early childhood education for exceptional children: A handbook of ideas and exemplary practices.* Reston, VA: Council for Exceptional Children.

Fixsen, D. L., Naoom, S. F., Blase, K. A., Freidman, R. M., & Wallace, F. (2005). *Implementation research: A synthesis of the literature.* Publication #231. Tampa, FL: University of South Florida, Louis de la Parte Florida Mental Health Institute, the National Implementation Research Network (FMHI).

Hebbeler, K., Smith, B. J., & Black, T. (1991). Federal early childhood special education policy: A model for the improvement of services for children with disabilities. *Exceptional Children, 58*(2), 104–112.

Hunt, J. M. (1961). *Intelligence and experience.* New York: Ronald Press.

Joyce, B., & Showers, B. (2002). *Student achievement through staff development* (3rd ed.). Alexandria, VA: Association for Supervision and Curriculum Development.

Mallory, B. (2007). Early childhood special education. In R. New & M. Cochran (Eds.), *Early childhood education: An international encyclopedia.* Westport, CT: Praeger.

New, R., & Cochran, M. (Eds.). (2007). *Early childhood education: An international encyclopedia.* Westport, CT: Praeger.

Sandall, S., Hemmeter, M., Smith, B., & McLean, M. (Eds.). (2005). *DEC recommended practices: A comprehensive guide for practical application.* Longmont, CO: Sopris West Publishing.

Shonkoff, J. P., & Meisels, S. J. (2003). *Handbook of early childhood intervention.* New York: Cambridge University Press.

Silverstein, R. (1988, February). A window of opportunity: P.L. 99-457. In *The intent and spirit of P.L. 99-457: A sourcebook.* Washington, DC: National Center for Clinical Infant Programs

Smith, B., & Bredekamp, S. (1998). Foreword. In L. Johnson, M. LaMontagne, P. Elgas, & A. Bauer (Eds.), *Early childhood education: Blending theory, blending practice.* Baltimore: Paul H. Brookes.

Smith, B., & Guralnick, M. (2007). Early intervention. In R. New & M. Cochran (Eds.), *Early childhood education: An international encyclopedia.* Westport, CT: Praeger.

Smith, B., Miller, P., & Bredekamp, S. (1998). Sharing responsibility: DEC-, NAEYC-, and Vygotsky-based practices for quality inclusion. *Young Exceptional Children, 2*(1), 11–20.

Smith, B. J. (1988). Early intervention public policy: Past, present, and future. In J. Jordan, J. J. Gallagher, R. J. Hutinger, & M. Karnes (Eds.), *Early childhood special education: Birth-three*. Reston, VA: Council for Exceptional Children.

Smith, B. J., & McKenna, P. (1994). Early intervention public policy: Past, present, and future. In L. Johnson, R. J. Gallagher, M. La Montagne, J. Jordan, J. J. Gallagher, P. Hutinger, & M. Karnes (Eds.), *Meeting early intervention challenges: Issues from birth to three*. Baltimore: Paul H. Brookes.

Weintraub, F., & Abeson, A. (1976). New education policies for the handicapped: The quiet revolution. In F. Weintraub, A. Abeson, J. Ballard, & M. LaVor (Eds.), *Public policy and the education of exceptional children*. Reston, VA: Council for Exceptional Children.

Chapter 2

Key National and State Policy Implementation Issues

Beth Rous and Barbara J. Smith

I n Chapter 1, historical trends in early intervention and early child-hood special education policies and issues were traced and described. This chapter builds on that history and describes current policies and issues for the field.

OVERVIEW OF FEDERAL SERVICES FOR YOUNG CHILDREN WITH SPECIAL NEEDS

As discussed in Chapter 1, there are three levels of government: federal, state, and local. At the federal level, the current system of services for young children has been described as diverse in terms of the focus of the various federal programs (Rous & Townley, 2010). For example, some programs are targeted to specific populations in an effort to prevent potential negative outcomes from known conditions (e.g., poverty is targeted by Head Start), while others are geared toward intervention due to existing conditions (e.g., Part C of IDEA). Some programs are universal in focus, including everyone (e.g., public school services), while still others are targeted (e.g., availability of child care to support working families). This section will provide specific information on major federal programs operated out of the U.S. Departments of Education, Health and Human Services, and Justice that impact young children with special needs, birth to age 8.

U.S. Department of Education

The Elementary and Secondary Education Act (ESEA, federal statute passed in 1965) provides federal support and guidance for elementary and secondary public school programs across the country. This statute, reauthorized every five years, has had several names. Most recently, it is named the No Child Left Behind Act of 2001. Funds through ESEA flow from the federal government to states, who then distribute funds to local school districts. ESEA does not mandate that states provide universal services to preschool-aged children, thus states who have public preschool programs have created and funded them on a voluntary basis. However, ESEA does include several programs to support vulnerable populations within schools. Those programs are extended to preschool populations served within the school. Examples include Title I, which provides compensatory education grants to schools and districts that focus on supporting students from low income families and improving their educational opportunities, and Title III, which focuses on supporting language instruction for students that have limited English proficiency (LEP).

In 2001, as part of the reauthorization of ESEA, a presidential initiative was created known as Good Start Grow Smart (GSGS). This initiative was designed to enhance accountability efforts in school-age programs (i.e., kindergarten through grade 12) by focusing on supporting high-quality early childhood programs across three main areas. First, GSGS called for strengthening Head Start programs through the development and implementation of a new accountability system that would emphasize early literacy development. Second, GSGS was designed to support states in enhancing early childhood quality, in part by supporting states in voluntarily establishing early learning guidelines for children ages three to five years. These guidelines are related to language and pre-reading skills. States are to align those guidelines with standards in place for K–12. Third, GSGS focused on improved access to research and evidence based practice for family members and professionals in the area of early childhood.

Within the Department of Education, the Office of Special Education Programs (OSEP) administers programs that fall under the Individuals with Disabilities Education Act (IDEA). Two specific components of IDEA relate to young children with disabilities. IDEA includes provisions for eligible children, birth to 3 years, to receive early intervention services. This is known as Part C of IDEA. Part C funds are distributed from the federal government to states. Under Part C, states have the option of designating a lead agency for services that vary across the Departments of Education, Health Services, or Human Services depending on the state. The lead agency is responsible for providing services to children who have a disability or are at substantial risk of developmental delay due to specific diagnosed conditions. States also have the option of serving children through Part C who have other risk conditions, such as biological/medical or environmental risk. The services under Part C are targeted to both the child and his or her family and are outlined in a document known as an Individualized Family Service Plan (IFSP). This IFSP is intended to be developed in partnership with the family by an interdisciplinary team of professionals. Every child and family is provided with a service coordinator or case manager to help coordinate services offered through the interdisciplinary team. For children in early intervention, IDEA provides provisions on the location of the services provided, indicating that these services must occur in the child's natural environment (e.g., home, child care program) to the maximum extent appropriate. Early intervention offers a range of services such as developmental and therapeutic services (e.g., physical, occupation and speech/language), family training and support, nutrition, and/or evaluation and assessment, depending on the child and family's level of need and as outlined in the IFSP.

IDEA also provides provisions for eligible children with disabilities ages 3 through 21 to receive a free appropriate public education (FAPE) through the public school system. This is known as Part B of IDEA. Part B funds flow from the federal level to state education agencies, who distribute them to local school districts. Within Part B, Section 619 specifically addresses the funding for services for preschool children (ages 3 to 5) who have a disability as determined by IDEA and each state's eligibility criteria. IDEA includes 14 disabilities definitions, including autism, deafness, deaf-blindness, emotional disturbance, hearing impairment, mental retardation, multiple disabilities, orthopedic impairment, other health impairment, specific learning disability, speech/language impairment, traumatic brain injury, and visual impairment. For children up to age 9, states may also use developmental delay as a category of eligibility. Once determined eligible, the specific special education and related services the child will receive are outlined in an Individualized Education Program (IEP). This plan is developed in collaboration with the family by a team that includes the child's regular education teacher, special education teacher, and other appropriate related services personnel such as the occupation, physical or speech/language therapist, mobility specialist, etc. Part B requires that the services a child receives are provided in the least restrictive environment (LRE). The goal of LRE is to support the inclusion of children with disabilities with their typically developing peers.

U.S. Department of Health and Human Services

One of the most well-known programs for young children is Head Start. In 1964, this comprehensive child development and family support program was established as part of the Economic Opportunity Act. The overall purpose of the program has been to support low-income families as a way to help break the cycle of poverty. The Head Start program is designed to serve 3- and 4-year-old children and includes a requirement to include children with disabilities (at least 10% of enrollment) in the program. During the reauthorization of 1994, Early Head Start programs were initiated. Early Head Start programs serve children up to age 3 and also include a 10 percent enrollment requirement for children with disabilities. Like ESEA and IDEA, the Head Start Act is reauthorized every five years. However, unlike programs through the Department of Education, Head Start funds are grant based and flow directly from the federal government to local grantees. Once funded, agencies are required to follow specific standards for program operation within the community(ies) they serve and are monitored through a regional network of offices.

In 1996, the Child Care and Development Block Grant (CCDBG), currently referred to as the Child Care and Development Fund (CCDF), was established. This block grant goes to states to support low-income working families in accessing child care through a subsidy program, as a way to support them in becoming and remaining independent. Within the CCDF statute, states are required to give priority to very-low-income families and those who have children with special needs. These funds also include provisions that focus on improving the quality of child care programs within states, as well as helping to ensure the availability of child care options.

Another long-standing program for young children is the Early and Periodic Screening, Diagnosis, and Treatment (EPSDT) program. EPSDT is a component of the Medicaid program and is designed to improve the health of low-income children. Services are mandated for children under the age of 18 who receive Medicaid and include periodic health checks, screening for physical and mental conditions (including dental, hearing, and vision), completing appropriate diagnostics tests if concerns are identified through screening, and providing appropriate treatment of such conditions. Another closely related program is the Children's Health Insurance Program (CHIP), which is administered by states and designed to provide health coverage for low-income families who are above the poverty cutoff for eligibility in Medicaid.

U.S. Department of Justice

The Americans with Disabilities Act (ADA) is a federal law designed to protect the civil rights of people with disabilities. This act, passed in 1990, prohibits discrimination against people with disabilities. The ADA has undergone numerous amendments since its passage and often has required review and interpretation through the court system (ADA, 2008). General provisions of the act require guarantees of equal opportunities for individuals with disabilities, including young children with special needs that are served in child care, Head Start, public schools, and other early childhood programs. Under Title III of ADA, early childhood programs, including private centers, generally cannot exclude children from programs due to their disability and must make reasonable modifications to policies and practices to support these children and make their facilities accessible.

KEY ISSUES IN THE FIELD

There are numerous issues facing the field of early intervention, including a move toward greater accountability for child outcomes, an emphasis on the use of evidence-based practice, and issues related to ensuring high-quality services and professionals who are qualified and trained to provide high-quality services. However, these issues must be considered within the context of the most pressing issue in our field—the continued desire to ensure that young children with special needs have the opportunity to participate in typical early childhood programs and services, or inclusion. Inclusion is not a new concept. It has been at the heart of early childhood special education legislation (e.g., natural environments, least restrictive environments) as well as other federal mandates in early childhood (e.g., Head Start and 10% disability enrollment requirements). Building on a joint position statement developed in 1993, in 2009, the Division for Early Childhood (DEC) of the Council for Exceptional Children (CEC) and the National Association for the Education of Young Children (NAEYC) proposed the following definition (DEC/NAEYC, 2009):

Early childhood inclusion embodies the values, policies, and practices that support the right of every infant and young child and his or her family, regardless of ability, to participate in a broad range of activities and contexts as full members of families, communities, and society. The desired results of inclusive experiences for children with and without disabilities and their families include a sense of belonging and membership, positive social relationships and friendships, and development and learning to reach their full potential. The defining features of inclusion that can be used to identify high quality early childhood programs and services are access, participation, and supports.

The development of this shared definition represents a defining moment in the fields of early intervention and early childhood as it provides clear guidelines that can positively influence research, policy, and practice. This definition includes three key components of inclusion that provide a framework for cross-sector work on increasing opportunities for inclusion for children of all abilities: (1) access; (2) participation, and (3) supports. From a policy perspective, several questions should be asked to determine the extent children have access to, can participate in, and have the supports needed to be successful in inclusive settings.

The first important question is: *Where do young children with special needs receive early intervention services, and to what extent are services provided in inclusive settings?* States report that 82 percent of those receiving early intervention services receive them in the home (Good, Lazara, & Danaher, 2008), 3.3 percent receive services in programs that serve typically developing children, while the remainder receive services in provider locations, such as clinics, hospitals, or residential facilities. Children and families are reported to receive on average between one and three hours a week of early intervention services (Hallam, Rous, Grove, & LoBianco, 2009; Kochanek & Buka, 1998; Shonkoff, Hauser-Cram, Krauss, Upshur, & Sameroff, 1992) and it is estimated that over half of children are in some type of nonparental care (e.g., child care, family, friend, or neighbor care) by nine months of age (Flanagan & West, 2004). At the preschool level, 25 percent of preschoolers with special needs receive their special education services in noninclusive settings (i.e., separate school, building, or residential facility), and only 48 percent spend at least 80 percent of their time in school with typically developing peers (Lazara, Dannaher, Kraus, & Goode, 2009).

The second question is: *How does the current structure of early childhood services in the United States support opportunities for inclusion for young children with special needs?* While there is a federal mandate to serve children with special needs (birth to 5 years), there is no federal mandate to offer general early childhood services and supports to typically developing children. Many states, however, do provide publicly supported preschool programs on a limited basis. Unlike school-age populations, publicly funded programs for infant-toddlers are generally designed on a home-visiting model, while publicly supported preschool programs (e.g., Head Start and public pre-kindergarten) are designed for targeted populations (i.e., economic risk, disability) and most often offered on a half-day (3 to 4 hours), part-week (e.g., 4-day versus 5-day) basis.

Therefore, children are likely to receive early childhood services in a combination of publicly and privately funded settings throughout a day. For example, an infant may be receiving early intervention services in the home for one hour a week, but is also enrolled in a child care program five days a week so that family members can work. A 3-year-old may spend four mornings a week in the public preschool program and the fifth day and each afternoon in a child care program. A 4-year-old of a single working parent may spend the early morning with family or a friend who drops them off at a Head Start center for the morning. The child is transported to the public preschool program in the afternoon, then to a child care program until the parent gets off work.

At the preschool level, funding of preschool programs designed to serve all children is left to state discretion. While there is considerable push on states to offer universal preschool services for 4-year olds, the National Institute for Early Education Research of the Department of Education (NIEER) reports that in 2008, 24 percent of 4-year olds and 3 percent of 3-year olds were served in state-funded preschool programs in the United States. Only three states make preschool services available for all 4-year olds, and no states are making universal services available for children under age 4 (Barnett, Epstein, Friedman, Boyd, & Hustedt, 2008). This provides a dilemma for states regarding how to provide inclusive settings. States and localities must collaborate across a variety of early childhood partners (e.g., Head Start, child care) to ensure that children are offered opportunities to participate with their nondisabled peers. Cross-agency collaboration requires communication, shared commitment to inclusion, supportive policies, and procedures in all agencies and professional development across agencies so that personnel can work together and share expertise related to meeting the educational needs of all children (Smith & Rose, 1993).

The third and most complex question is: *How can we ensure that services provided in inclusive settings are of high quality and meet the needs of children with special needs?* While the concept of inclusion is not new, the actual practice of including children with special needs in a variety of early childhood programs remains difficult. There have been numerous efforts over the last two decades to provide targeted support to programs in supporting children with a variety of needs in typical early childhood settings. Some have been focused on research (e.g., Early Childhood Research Institute on Inclusion) and some on professional development (e.g., Special Quest, Head Start Center for Inclusion, and National Professional Development Center on Inclusion).

Recently, there has been a growing recognition that to increase the inclusion of children in early childhood settings, we must focus attention on embedding these efforts within the national initiatives to improve overall quality in early care and education settings. In other words, included children with special needs in poor-quality settings will not produce the kinds of overall outcomes that are possible. The broader early childhood field has a long history of efforts to address the quality of child-care settings (Rous & Townley, 2010). However, the last decade has seen a dramatic increase of state-level efforts to develop Quality Rating and Improvement Systems (QRIS) and other initiatives that include specific standards of quality related to program structure and the environments in which children spend time (e.g., National Association for the Education of Young Children [NAEYC], 2005). Others focus on adult-child/child-child interactions within those environments (e.g., Pianta & Hamre, 2009). These efforts within states have primarily focused on child care programs. Commonly accepted elements of quality initiatives in early care and education settings include (1) program standards, (2) accountability measures, (3) program and practitioner outreach and support, (4) financial incentives, and (5) parent education (Child Care Bureau, 2007). Although child care programs serve young children with disabilities, few states have explicitly included standard or elements related to children with special needs (Child Care Bureau, 2007; Hallam, Rous, & Cox, 2008).

Another aspect of quality includes the increasing emphasis on the use of evidence-based (also referred to as scientifically or research-based) practice. This has required renewed efforts to define high-quality research, identify specific practices that have a research evidence base, and identify processes by which providers and teachers can choose appropriate instructional and curricular approaches for implementation. Of particular importance for children with special needs is the ability to implement these practices in inclusive settings. The Institute for Educational Sciences (IES) in the U.S. Department of Education supports this goal by providing specific research priorities that focus on identifying new interventions (Goal 2), determining the impact of these interventions (Goal 3), and exploring the large-scale implementation of interventions in a variety of settings (Goal 4; IES, 2009).

Professional development plays a critical role in the implementation of evidence-based practice to support children in inclusive settings. As proposed by Buysse, Winton, and Rous (2009), professional development means using evidence-based strategies to facilitate "teaching and learning experiences that are transactional and designed to support the acquisition of professional knowledge, skills, and dispositions as well as the application of this knowledge in practice" (p. 239). These professional development efforts include those focused on training at the pre-service (e.g., 2- and 4-year colleges and universities) and in-service level (national and regional training networks), as well as technical assistance services. Training and technical assistance providers also have the responsibility to use evidence-based practice in the design and delivery of training and technical assistance services as well as support practitioners and programs in identifying evidence-based practices for implementation across settings. They must know which practices are effective and how to teach them to providers so that they can implement them appropriately in their work setting. The challenge for states is to fund and support such effective technical assistance networks. As Blasé (2009) points out, the adoption of evidence-based practices requires on-site coaching and support.

Finally, the development of specific accountability measures within early childhood systems can impact the level to which children with special needs are included in programs with typically development children and the degree to which their individual needs are supported in these environments. Accountability for results is not a new idea in the area of early childhood special education. Monitoring systems at the state and local level have been in place since the passage of Public Law 99-457 in 1986. However, passage of the Government Performance Results Act (GPRA) in 1993 has led to increased accountability demands across all sectors of the federal government through requirements to document stated results from programs (Harbin, Rous, & McLean, 2005). Through GPRA, Congress requires federal agencies to identify specific goals for each program they administer, establish indicators for those programs, and beginning in 2002, participate in Program Assessment Rating Tool (PART). PART is an assessment process developed and implemented through the Office of Management and Budget (OMB) to determine the degree to which program results can be demonstrated. This process was designed to align the GPRA process with budget decisions.

The increased emphasis on accountability includes results at the child/student level. This is evidenced by new requirements for increased student achievement in ESEA and measuring impact of programs on specific child outcomes in Head Start, early intervention, and early childhood special education. For example, in early intervention and early childhood special education, OSEP requires state-level aggregate data on the degree to which children participating in IDEA Part C and Part B, §619 have met three specific child outcomes. These outcomes are designed to measure children's progress against typically developing peers in (1) positive social-emotional skills, (2) acquisition and use of knowledge and skills, and (3) use of appropriate behaviors to meet their needs (Hebbeler & Barton, 2007).

EARLY INTERVENTION POLICY WITHIN THE BROADER EARLY CHILDHOOD SYSTEM

The last two decades have seen significant growth in services provided to young children in the United States, both with and without disabilities, through public school preschool, Head Start, and child care programs. Despite tough economic times, the National Conference of State Legislators reported increased funding of early childhood efforts during 2009 (Poppe & Clothier, 2009).This expansion of public and private early childhood programs may be attributed to two major factors. First, the number of dual- and single-parent families in the workforce has increased dramatically, which in turn has increased the need for out-of-home care for working families. Second, research findings have led to a better understanding of the relationship between high-quality early childhood experiences and later school and life success (e.g., Gormley, Phillips, & Gayer, 2008; Shonkoff & Phillips, 2000; Wong, Cook, Barnett, & Jung, 2008).

As discussed earlier in this chapter, the number and type of programs for young children is diverse, with program administration across a number of federal and state agencies. With the increased support for early childhood programs, there has also been a renewed focus on ensuring various federal and state programs for young children engage in more collaborative efforts. Interestingly, the push for collaboration across programs has shifted in terms of the primary initiators of the collaborative efforts. In the late 1980s and early 1990s, there were several initiatives in early childhood special education to bring other "early childhood partners" to the table to support the inclusion of young children with special needs in their programs and services. This was especially crucial in the area of transition of young children into school programs (e.g., Rosenkoetter, Hains, & Fowler, 1994; Rous, Hemmeter, & Schuster, 1994). More recently, there have been increased efforts to support "cross-sector" collaboration by early childhood educators. These efforts have been spurred by recognition of the increasing diversity of young children (e.g., cultural, ethnic, language, and ability) in public preschool, Head Start, and child care programs and the need to provide specific supports and expertise to these programs for meeting these diverse needs (Smith, Miller, & Bredekamp, 1998).

These efforts have received significant support at the federal level through the Early Learning Challenge Fund initiative (U.S. Department of Education, 2009), which focuses on supporting states in developing more integrated and collaborative systems for early learning across states. This focus on cross-sector collaboration was combined with the growth of early care, intervention, and education programs across the country. The initiative is designed to provide new opportunities at the state and local levels to engage in meaningful dialogue around critical issues for children with special needs within the broader early childhood systems. This is seen as especially important, given the fragmented nature of the early care, intervention, and education system in the United States. There is a need to ensure the inclusion of young children with disabilities in all aspects of these systems, including professional development, quality initiatives such as state Quality Rating and Improvement systems and program standards, and accountability efforts such as child outcome reporting, state data systems, and early learning guidelines/standards (Buysse & Hollingsworth, 2009). The specific components included in the proposed 2009 Early Learning Challenge Fund can be used as a framework for these important conversations (as outlined in Table 2.1).

Table 2.1   Key Considerations for Children with Special Needs within the Broader Early Childhood System Components

Early Learning Challenge Fund Component[1]	Key Issues or Considerations for Children with Special Needs
Aligned early learning and development standards that lead to school readiness and are integrated with program quality to guide curriculum and program development	• Representativeness of a range of ability levels in standards including children who have significant and/or multiple disabilities • Consideration for developmental patterns of young children with disabilities and the range of environments in which young children with disabilities are served • Linkages between evidence-based practice and intervention strategies that have been proven effective for young children with disabilities
An evidence-based quality rating system structured with progressive levels of quality—which may be used across early learning settings and programs	• Needs of young children with disabilities are explicitly addressed in Quality Rating and Improvement Systems (QRIS) standards • Range of physical, social, and developmental needs of children with special needs are addressed • Program standards developed by professional associations for children with special needs included and referenced (e.g., Division for Early Childhood; Occupational Therapy Association) are referenced
An effective system of program review, monitoring, and improvement applied across all programs and settings	• Indicators required for state monitoring through the Office of Special Education Programs (OSEP) are integrated within the system
An evidence-based system of professional development to prepare an effective and well-qualified workforce of early educators, including appropriate levels of training, education, and credentials	• Guidelines/standards and evidence-based practices are embedded across professional development activities implemented at both the preservice and in-service levels across systems • Needs of providers serving children with special needs are considered in core content across settings

(Continued)

Table 2.1   (Continued)

Early Learning Challenge Fund Component[1]	Key Issues or Considerations for Children with Special Needs
Strategies for families and parents to better assess quality in their child's early learning program and better support their child's learning	• QRIS systems include specific information on programs that provide inclusive services for children across a range of disabilities
Systems to facilitate screening and referrals for health, mental health, disability, and family support	• Systems are in place to reduce duplication of effort in screening and diagnosis of children with disabilities based on eligibility criteria
A coordinated zero-to-five data infrastructure to collect essential information on where young children spend their time and the effectiveness of programs that serve them	• The needs of children with a range of disabilities is considered in the identification of assessments and measures • The multiple environments in which children may be concurrently served is considered in development of data systems
An age- and developmentally appropriate curriculum and assessment system that is used to guide practice, improve programs, and inform kindergarten readiness	• Recommended practices related to curriculum and assessment developed by professional associations for children with special needs are included and referenced (e.g., Division for Early Childhood; Occupational Therapy Association)

[1]Components are presented at: http://www2.ed.gov/about/inits/ed/earlylearning/elcf -factsheet.html.

LEADERSHIP IMPLICATIONS AND RECOMMENDATIONS FOR POLICY AND PRACTICE

State and local leaders play a critical role in designing and implementing early intervention service structures that support the inclusion of young children with special needs. Given the current context of cross-sector services and supports, those in leadership positions have an obligation to seek, understand, and implement evidence-based leadership skills. However, many times, leaders in the field of early childhood rise to leadership positions through their content knowledge in early childhood and/or basic managerial skills without the benefit of professional development in the area of leadership.

Hundreds of books, articles, and documents provide definitions and descriptions of quality leadership (e.g., Bolman & Deal, 2008; Covey, 1991). Definitions of good leaders have been provided across disciplines (e.g., business, education) and typically take the form of descriptions of the qualities, skills, or competencies that leaders must have. Leaders are defined as either effective or ineffective. Kagan and Bowman (1997) defined the role of leadership in early childhood programs by presenting five dimensions of leadership: (1) pedagogical, (2) administrative, (3) advocacy, (4) community, and (5) conceptual. These dimensions provide a general framework, but do not differentiate between administration/management, which involves the day-to-day operation of a program, and leadership, which involves an ability to influence stakeholders towards accomplishing organizational goals.

The U.S. Department of Education identified five dimensions of leadership key to sustain reform efforts that can provide insights for today's early childhood leaders (U.S. Department of Education, 1996) to make significant progress within the context of today's cross-sector early childhood environment, especially toward a goal of ensuring more inclusive opportunities for young children, a report on leadership, and school reform. These dimensions include (1) partnership and voice; (2) vision and values; (3) knowledge and daring; (4) savvy and persistence; and (5) recognition that personal qualities such as passion, humor, and empathy play a role in effective leadership. The first, *partnership and voice*, involves the ability of early childhood leaders to gather information from a wide variety of stakeholders and include those stakeholders in all aspects of the program. The second dimension, *vision and values*, requires early childhood leaders to be clear about the vision for early childhood services and to work with other partners to keep that vision alive by working in partnership to sustain the values that support it. Third, *knowledge and daring* requires leaders to be willing and able to take risks, such as implementing a new curriculum or technology. However, they need to be able to balance this risk-taking so that risks are calculated based on the development and sustenance of evidence-based practice and emerging knowledge in the field. Fourth, being *savvy and persistent* involves leaders having an understanding of how the system works and the ability to promote cooperation across the system. To this list, we would add the important characteristics associated with effective collaborative leadership. As noted earlier, the early childhood world is comprised of many early childhood and early intervention systems and programs that need to work together to ensure all children's and families' needs are met and effective inclusive services are available to children with disabilities. This requires that programs work together to build a unified system (Hayden, Frederick, & Smith, 2003).

The current approach to building leaders in the field of early intervention, as well as early childhood, needs focused attention. As the interest in supporting early childhood programs continues to grow, the field must shift from an on-the-job training model to a more coordinated and planned approach to identifying what early childhood leaders need to know to be effective and providing clear pathways for building leaders and ensuring they have acquired those competencies, knowledge, and skills. The current approach in early childhood stands in contrast other comparable fields, like education, in which there are clear delineations of the skills and competencies required for school leaders. Through the Interstate School Leaders Licensure Consortium (ISLLC), six standards (Figure 2.1) were designed to reflect current research in educational leadership and provide a framework for research, policy, and practice, as well as professional

Figure 2.1   ISLLC Educational Leadership Policy Standards

1. An education leader promotes the success of every student by facilitating the development, articulation, implementation, and stewardship of a vision of learning that is shared and supported by all stakeholders.
2. An education leader promotes the success of every student by advocating, nurturing, and sustaining a school culture and instructional program conducive to student learning and staff professional growth.
3. An education leader promotes the success of every student by ensuring management of the organization, operation, and resources for a safe, efficient, and effective learning environment.
4. An education leader promotes the success of every student by collaborating with faculty and community members, responding to diverse community interests and needs, and mobilizing community resources.
5. An education leader promotes the success of every student by acting with integrity, fairness, and in an ethical manner.
6. An education leader promotes the success of every student by understanding, responding to, and influencing the political, social, economic, legal, and cultural context.

development and credential systems for educational leaders (Council of Chief State School Officers, 2008).

Following a similar model in early childhood special education would require rethinking our current certification and credentialing systems to embed leadership content particularly at the master's and doctoral level. Identifying key knowledge, skills, and competencies constitutes the first steps. One such effort in this area was Project Lead, a leadership grant funded through the United States Department of Education, Office of Special Education Programs (OSEP). Through this project, a set of early intervention–early childhood leadership competencies were developed that were aligned with the ISLLC standards (Harbin, Neal, & Malloy, 2003). These standards include knowledge, dispositions, and practices across seven leadership dimensions: pedagogical, organizational, human resources, collaborative, political, systems, and symbolic.

Designing more explicit leadership standards and programs can help us support leaders better able to address ongoing issues in the field of early intervention at the system level. They will be able to respond to the changing political context. They will be responsive to current research and contribute to a research agenda that can focus on broader issues that affect policy and practice. For example, currently in early intervention, we have divergent structures at the state levels for services for infants and toddlers (e.g., vendor versus agency-based systems; primary versus team-based provider models; dedicated versus primary service coordination; Good, Lazara, & Danaher, 2008). However, little attention has been paid to the effectiveness, advantages, and disadvantages of these structures. These are key policy issues that need to be addressed if we are to build an effective system of services for young children with disabilities and their families.

REFERENCES

Americans with Disabilities Act (ADA). (2008). Sec. 3406. Retrieved from http://frwebgate.access.gpo.gov/cgi-bin/getdoc.cgi?dbname=110_cong_bills&docid=f:s3406enr.txt.pdf

Barnett, W. S., Epstein, D. J, Friedman, A. H., Boyd, J. S., & Hustedt, J. T. (2008). *The state of preschool: 2008 state preschool yearbook.* New Brunswick, NJ: National Institute for Early Education Research.

Blasé, K. (2009). Technical assistance to promote service and system change. *Roadmap to Effective Intervention Practices #4.* Tampa, FL: University of South Florida, Technical Assistance Center on Social Emotional Intervention for Young Children.

Bolman, L. G., & Deal, T. E. (2008). *Reframing organizations: Artistry, choice and leadership* (4th ed.). San Francisco: Jossey-Bass.

Buysse, V., & Hollingsworth, H. L. (2009). Program quality and early childhood inclusion: Recommendations for professional development. *Topics in Early Childhood Special Education 29*(2), 119–128.

Buysse, V., Winton, P., & Rous, B. (2009). Reaching consensus on a definition of professional development for the early childhood field. *Topics in Early Childhood Special Education 28*(4), 235–243.

Child Care Bureau (2007). *Child care bulletin 32: Systemic approaches to improving quality of care QRS gain ground across the nation.* Washington, DC: Author.

Council of Chief State School Officers (2008). *Educational leadership policy standards: ISLLC 2008 as adopted by the national policy board for educational administration.* Washington, DC: Author.

Covey, S. R. (1991). *Principle-centered leadership.* New York: Simon & Schuster.

DEC/NAEYC. (2009). Early childhood inclusion: A joint position statement of the Division for Early Childhood (DEC) and the National Association for the Education of Young Children (NAEYC). Chapel Hill: University of North Carolina, FPG Child Development Institute.

Flanagan, K., & West, J. (2004). Children born in 2001: First results from the base year of the Early Childhood Longitudinal Study, Birth Cohort (ECLS-B). NCES 2005-036. Washington, DC: National Center for Education Statistics. Retrieved from http://www.childcareresearch.org/childcare/resources/4623/pdf

Goode, S., Lazara, A., & Danaher, J. (Eds.). (2008). Part C updates (10th ed.). Chapel Hill: University of North Carolina, FPG Child Development Institute, National Early Childhood Technical Assistance Center.

Gormley, W. T., Phillips, D., & Gayer, T. (2008). Preschool programs can boost school readiness. *Science, 27*(320), 1723–1724.

Hallam, R., Rous, B., & Cox, M. (2008, February). Quality child care for young children with disabilities: An examination of statewide child care quality rating systems. Poster session presented at the Conference on Research Innovations in Early Intervention, San Diego, CA.

Hallam, R., Rous, B., Grove, J., & LoBianco, T. (2009). Level and intensity of early intervention services for infants and toddlers with disabilities. *Journal of Early Intervention, 31*(2), 179–196.

Harbin, G., Neal, P., & Malloy, W. (2003). *Early childhood leadership competencies.* Project LEAD. Chapel Hill: University of North Carolina, FPG Child Development Institute.

Harbin, G., Rous, B., & McLean, M. (2005). Feature article: Issues in designing state accountability systems. *Journal of Early Intervention, 27*(3), 137–164.

Hayden, P., Frederick, L., & Smith, B. J. (2003). *A roadmap for facilitating collaborative teams.* Longmont, CO: Sopris West Publishing.

Hebbeler, K., & Barton, L. (2007). The need for data on child and family outcomes at the federal and state levels. *Young Exceptional Children Monograph Series, 9,* 1–15.

Institute for Educational Sciences (IES), U.S. Department of Education. (2009). Preparing an application. Retrieved from http://ies.ed.gov/funding/prep.asp

Kagan, S. L., & Bowman, B. (1997). *Leadership in early care and education.* Washington, DC: National Association for the Education of Young Children.

Kochanek, T. T., & Buka, S. L. (1998). Patterns of service utilization: Child, maternal, and service provider factors. *Journal of Early Intervention, 21*(3), 217–231.

Lazara, A., Danaher, J., Kraus, R., & Goode, S. (Eds.). (2009). *Section 619 Profile* (16th ed.). Chapel Hill: University of North Carolina, FPG Child Development Institute, National Early Childhood Technical Assistance Center.

National Association for the Education of Young Children (NAEYC). (2005). Position statements of NAEYC. Retrieved from http://www.naeyc.org/position statements

Pianta, R., & Hamre, B. K. (2009). Classroom processes and positive youth development: Conceptualizing, measuring, and improving the capacity of interactions between teachers and students. *New Directions for Youth Development, 121,* 33–46.

Poppe, J., & Clothier, S. (2009). *Early care and education state budget actions FY 2009.* Denver, CO: National Conference of State Legislatures.

Rosenkoetter, S. E., Hains, A. H., & Fowler, S. A. (1994). *Bridging early services for children with special needs and their families: A practical guide for transitioning planning.* Baltimore: Paul H. Brookes.

Rous, B., Hemmeter, M. L., & Schuster, J. (1994). Sequenced transition to education in the public schools: A systems approach to transition planning. *Topics in Early Childhood Special Education 14*(3).

Rous, B., & Townley, K. F. (2010). Early childhood policy and implications for quality initiatives. In P. Wesley & V. Buysse (Eds.), *The quest for quality: Promising innovations for early childhood programs.* Baltimore: Paul H. Brookes.

Shonkoff, J. P., Hauser-Cram, P., Krauss, M. W., Upshur, C. C., & Sameroff, A. J. (1992). *Development of infants with disabilities and their families: Implications for theory and service delivery.* Monographs of the Society for Research in Child Development.

Shonkoff, J., & Phillips, D. A. (Eds.). (2000). *From neurons to neighborhoods: The science of early childhood development.* Washington, DC: National Academy Press, National Research Council and Institute of Medicine.

Smith, B., Miller, P., & Bredekamp, S. (1998). Sharing responsibility: DEC-, NAEYC-, and Vygotsky-based practices for quality inclusion. *Young Exceptional Children, 2*(1), 11–20.

Smith, B. J., & Rose, D. F. (1993). *The administrator's policy handbook for preschool mainstreaming.* Cambridge, MA: Brookline Books, Inc.

U.S. Department of Education. (1996). *The role of leadership in sustaining school reform: Voices from the field.* Washington, DC.

U.S. Department of Education. (2009). *The Early Learning Challenge Fund.* Retrieved from http://www2.ed.gov/about/inits/ed/earlylearning/elcf-factsheet.html

Wong, V. C., Cook, T. D., Barnett, W. S., & Jung, K. (2008). An effectiveness-based evaluation of five state pre-kindergarten programs. *Journal of Policy Analysis and Management, 27*(1), 122–154.

Chapter 3

Early Intervention: International Policies and Programs

Joan C. Eichner, Christina Groark, and Oleg Palmov

In our globalized society, it is important to understand early intervention as it is implemented and interpreted around the world. This chapter reviews the international political and practice environments for serving young children who are at risk of developing disabilities or have diagnosed disabilities. It describes international laws, conventions, and agreements that cover the rights of children with disabilities and the policies and practices that provide support and services to these populations in a diverse sample of countries. These countries include Canada, Russia, China, New Zealand, Brazil, and South Africa.

CHILD RIGHTS–BASED INTERNATIONAL POLICIES

A common definition is useful to analyze global policies on disability. According to the Convention on the Right of Persons with Disabilities, Article 1: "Persons with disabilities include those who have long-term physical, mental, intellectual, or sensory impairment which in interaction with various barriers may hinder their full and effective participation in society on an equal basis with others" (prepared by UN Web Services Section, Department of Public Information, United Nations, 2006). However, the definition used in each country varies. Often there may be no universally agreed-upon definition, or the definitions of disability may vary among a country's policies. For purposes of this chapter, we follow the standard of the Convention of the Rights of the Child, which outlines the human rights entitlements of all children, regardless of their abilities.

THE CONVENTION ON THE RIGHTS OF THE CHILD

The 1989 Convention on the Rights of the Child (CRC) sets a human-rights standard by which to judge the treatment of, and services for, children in all countries. To date, 193 countries have ratified the CRC. Every member of the United Nations (UN) has ratified it except the United States and Somalia (United Nations Children's Fund [UNICEF], 2008). The CRC identifies minimum political, civil, social, and economic rights to which all children are entitled. These rights are considered by the CRC to be essential, universally accepted, and nonnegotiable by any government. Governments that support the CRC share responsibility to ensure the rights of all children are guarded and respected. The CRC is based on four principles: Nondiscrimination; devotion to the best interests of the child; the right to life, survival, and development; and respect for the views of the child. The CRC is the first globally recognized legal document that focuses on the unique needs and vulnerabilities of individuals under age 18.

The CRC recognizes that a supportive and nurturing environment is essential for a child to develop to his or her fullest potential, and this environment is created by social, cultural, political, economic, and civil rights (United Nations Educational, Scientific and Cultural Organization [UNESCO], 2009). Articles 27–29 require countries that have pledged support to the CRC to recognize a child's right to basic education at an appropriate level for the child, and a standard of living that is sufficient to allow the child to develop physically, mentally, spiritually, morally, and socially (UNICEF, 2008).

Article 23 of the CRC pertains to children with special needs. Part I assures that governments accepting the CRC recognize and protect the basic rights of children with disabilities and ensure their full and active participation in society. Part II states that any child with special needs should be informed of, and receive, appropriate care and services, subject to available resources. Part III removes financial barriers to care by stating that assistance should be provided to families at no cost, whenever possible, while "taking into account the financial resources of the parents or others caring for the child." This covers education, health care, rehabilitation, employment training and assistance, recreation, and cultural, social, and spiritual development opportunities. Part IV of Article 23 states that all countries supporting the CRC should openly share knowledge and best practices, with the intention of enhancing the capacity of under-resourced countries (United Nations

Office of the High Commissioner for Human Rights [UNOHCHR], 1990; UNICEF, 2008).

The CRC may be either supported or ratified. Countries that support it express a commitment to recognize and protect children's human rights. Countries that ratify the CRC are legally bound by the United Nations and the other supporting countries to uphold their commitment; however, the specific policies and practices used in each nation are subject to that country's need and interpretation. All actions that supporting or ratifying countries undertake must be in the best interests of children.

The CRC is significant because it represents a global promise to recognize and protect the rights of all children. However, it also acknowledges the challenges some countries may face as they attempt to meet the needs of children with disabilities. These challenges may stem from limited economic resources, a lack of trained professionals, public stigma, superstitions or misinformation about disabilities, political unwillingness, or other reasons. CRC is useful as a rallying tool that establishes global goals for advocates and supporters of children with all types of special needs. It focuses attention on the issues affecting these children and the commitment all countries should make to advance their quality of life. However, the CRC does not require or guarantee a supporting country will implement steps to achieve these goals. Each country that subscribes to the convention must consider how it can meet the CRC goals given its unique population and economic, political, and social contexts.

OTHER INTERNATIONAL POLICIES INFLUENCING CHILD RIGHTS

International legislation specific to early intervention is rare; however, the principle of universal human rights can be used to judge the policies and programs offered in individual countries. The following policies that frame education, health care, and access to equal public services as human rights show an evolution in international laws and regulations that affect children with disabilities.

The 1948 Universal Declaration of Human Rights, Article 25(2), recognizes childhood as a time that merits special care, assistance, and protection (United Nations, 1948). Acceptance of the Universal Declaration shows political support for equality for all people of all countries, ethnicities, genders, religions, and socioeconomic backgrounds who should be respected for their essential worth as human beings. A state that accepts the Universal Declaration chooses to become legally obligated by it, and the United Nations has established mechanisms that hold governments accountable for human-rights violations.

Many international policies regarding children focus on their right to education. In the forward to *A Human Rights Based Approach to Education for All*, Vernor Muñoz, UN Special Rapporteur on the Right to Education, describes education as the primary vehicle by which economically and socially marginalized adults and children can lift themselves out of poverty and obtain the means to participate fully in their communities (UNICEF, 2007). Similar statements appear in such treaties as the United Nations Educational, Scientific, and Cultural Organization's (UNESCO) Convention against Discrimination in Education (1960), the International Covenant on Economic, Social, and Cultural Rights (1966), and the United Nations Convention on the Rights of the Child (1989) (UNICEF, 2007). These policies show the international community that education is a human entitlement to which children with special needs should not be excluded; indeed, education may be the only available vehicle through which vulnerable or marginalized children can achieve a better quality of life.

One policy specific to children with disabilities is the "Declaration on the Rights of Disabled Persons" (the Declaration) adopted by the United Nations General Assembly (UNGA) in 1975. The Declaration describes the rights of persons with disabilities to receive services tailored to their particular needs, the right to appropriate treatments, and the right to environments and living conditions that are appropriate but are as equivalent as possible to those of their contemporaries. The Declaration also promotes integration of mixed-ability individuals, thereby representing a philosophical shift towards inclusion (United Nations, 1975; World Health Organization, 2005; World Health Organization Regional Office for Europe, 2005). The UNGA went on to establish 1981 as the International Year of Disabled Persons, a move that emphasized global public awareness, disability prevention, rehabilitation, and equal opportunities for all (United Nations Enable Convention on the Rights of Persons with Disabilities, 1976). The year led to the formation of the World Program of Action Concerning Disabled Persons (WPA), adopted in 1982. The WPA is a global strategy to prevent disabilities, improve rehabilitation, and equalize opportunities. Like its predecessors, the WPA frames equality for individuals with disabilities as a human-rights issue that requires national, regional, and international action and support (United Nations Enable, 1982).

In 1990, a global commitment to education was renewed by representatives from over 300 countries and nongovernmental organizations in Jomtien, Thailand, at the World Conference on Education for All. The resulting Jomtien Declaration on Education for All extended the right of basic education to early childhood by affirming that learning begins at birth and that early childhood care and education (ECCE) is an integral part of basic education. It recognized that ECCE should be provided in multiple settings, including the home and community (Article 5). The Jomtien Declaration cites children's rights and needs for educational opportunities to develop academic skills and the values, attitudes, knowledge, and skills they will need to survive and thrive into adulthood. The Jomtien Declaration pays special attention to vulnerable groups such as children with disabilities (UNESCO, 2009). The Jomtien Declaration was supported in 1993, the 48th session of the UNGA, which adopted the Standard Rules on Equalization Opportunities for Persons with Disabilities. This agreement is not legally binding, but the Standard Rules are used as a policy-making tool and establish a political and moral commitment to achieve equal opportunities for individuals with special needs. Several of the Standard Rules impact young children with special needs and mirror aspects of the modern early intervention model. For example, Rule Two outlines the need for states to provide multidisciplinary professional teams for the early detection, assessment, and treatment. Rule Three focuses on appropriate rehabilitation techniques that ensure the full and equal participation of the individual in society. Rule Six recognizes that very young children and preschool-aged children need special consideration in education through inclusive, culturally sensitive, and appropriate pedagogy designed to meet individualized needs (United Nations Enable, 1993).

International support for child rights continued throughout the 1990s. In 1994, over 300 representatives from 92 governments and 25 international organizations met in Salamanca, Spain, under the auspices of UNESCO, to further the objective of Education for All. The Conference adopted the Salamanca Statement on Principles, Policy, and Practice in Special Needs Education and a Framework for Action. These documents highlight the principles of inclusion and recognize the need to work toward schools that include all children, embrace differences, support learning, and respond to individual children's needs. This step was an important contribution to the goal of achieving Education for All and sets a standard for inclusive and equal services. UNESCO's 2009 report, *Policy Guidelines on Inclusion in Education*, is an update on the movement toward inclusive education, a major step toward universal education for all children. This document defines inclusive education broadly, discusses its educational and social value and cost-effectiveness, and identifies challenges to designing and implementing inclusive education systems (UNESCO, 2009).

In April 2000, over 1,000 people from 164 countries attended the World Education Forum in Dakar, Senegal, and ultimately adopted the Dakar Framework for Action, Education for All. The Dakar Framework affirms a right to free and compulsory primary education for all children regardless of limited resources in their home country (paragraph 10). This represented a step forward because participating countries dedicated themselves to expansion and improvement of early childhood care and education with particular focus on the most "vulnerable and disadvantaged children" (paragraph 7; UNESCO, 2009). In late 2007, UNESCO published *Education for All Global Monitoring Report* on global progress toward meeting the universal education goals that were outlined in 2000. This report indicates a significant increase in primary school enrollment, from 647 million in 1999 to 688 million in 2005. Despite this progress, more than 50 countries will not meet the goal of universal primary education by 2015, and gender disparity in attendance of primary school remains a global program. Furthermore, the focus on improving primary education has overshadowed efforts in early childhood education despite research supporting the importance of investing in this crucial early period of a child's development (UNESCO, 2007).

The last major international policy covered here, the Convention on the Rights of Persons with Disabilities (the Convention) and its Optional Protocol (a related document that outlines procedures that may be used by countries adopting the Convention), was adopted in December 2006 by the United Nations. It is the first comprehensive human rights treaty of the twenty-first century and reflects the evolution from viewing persons with disabilities as charity recipients to accepting them as individuals who are knowledgeable of their rights, capable of claiming those rights, and active members of society.

Each of the policies described here outlines principles that countries should strive to follow and not contradict through national-level laws or actions. The policies have wide-ranging goals with vast differences in implementation and the level of achievement reached in supporting countries. Some of them include qualifications, such as being subject to available resources, which provide countries a necessary means to show support, but not meet, the ideal described by international standards. Even with their limitations, these policies are advantageous because they draw global attention and coordination action to meet the educational, health, social and other needs of all children. Countries that represent every geographic area of the world were chosen to illustrate how each country has interpreted and implemented global- and national-level policies. Although executed in disparate cultures, political contexts, and economic conditions, all of the efforts described in this chapter seek to improve the health, well-being, and education of all children with unique and diverse needs.

COUNTRIES

Canada

Background and Demographics

At 3.8 million square miles, Canada is the world's second-largest country physically. It is a highly developed industrial society with a population of 33.5 million. The majority of the population is of British, French, or other European descent, while smaller percentages of people identify with Amerindian, Asian, African, Arab, or mixed background (United States Central Intelligence Agency, 2009b). Overall, Canadians enjoy a high quality of life, long life expectancy, and a low infant mortality rate (United States Department of State, 2008).

Each of Canada's provinces (similar to states in the United States) and territories administer child care services that typically include preschools, center-based child care, and regulated family child care. These jurisdictions are also responsible for kindergarten starting at age 5. While kindergarten is seen as a public responsibility, preschool services for children under age 5 are viewed as a private matter. There is a wide range in quality, type, and availability of early childhood services among Canada's regions, and it is generally agreed that no region has a model system that meets the needs of most children and families (Friendly, 2007).

Key Early Intervention Issues and Prevalence

The prevalence of early childhood disability is difficult to measure because of delayed diagnosis and underreporting, but it is estimated that there are 26,210 Canadian children with special needs between birth and age 4 (Max Bell Foundation, 2006). The majority of these children are classified with a "delay," followed by hearing and vision impairments (McGill University & Yaldei Development Center, 2006). The Canadian Human Resources and Skills Development program's 2008 report *Advancing the Inclusion of People with Disabilities* states that the disability rate has increased from 12.4 percent in 2001 to 14.3 percent in 2006 (affecting approximately 4,417,870 individuals in 2006). Most of this increase is due to an aging population; however, the rate of childhood learning disabilities also increased significantly (Government of Canada, 2008).

National Early Intervention Policies and Programs

Canada now has federal legislation specific to disabilities, leaving many of Canada's provinces to enact their own policy and practice (Burns and Gordon, 2009). The national government, particularly the Department of Justice and the Canadian Human Rights Commission, promotes and supports the rights of individuals with disabilities to social inclusion and active participation in society through a number of initiatives and a comprehensive legal framework. In the 1980s, the government enacted the Canadian Charter of Rights and Freedoms (1982) and the Canadian Human Rights Act (1985), legal measures to protect equal rights and freedom from discrimination for all, including discrimination based on physical or mental disabilities (Government of Canada, 2008). Canada supported human rights globally by drafting the United Nations Convention of the Rights of Persons with Disabilities (Government of Canada, 2008). It has also made a commitment to increasing community living, but each of the 13 provinces and territories of Canada retain individual choice about institutionalization. Currently, British Columbia, Ontario, and Newfoundland have closed all their institutions. However, other provinces and territories are actively funding and building them (S. Rattai, personal communication, January 12, 2010).

Canada has a number of national policies that support prevention or amelioration of developmental delays and disability in young children through poverty reduction and family support. Physical and mental health and social assistance services are viewed as part of the larger system of economic and social supports provided to Canadian families. Children's preventative health services are supported by a national health system and insurance plan. Children receive well-baby services by the family's primary care physician and free home-visiting programs that are provided to all families. Mothers, and to some extent fathers, receive six months of paid leave from employment around the birth of a child (Kamerman, 2000).

In 2000, the national government agreed to provide $500 million Canadian per year to provinces and territories to improve and expand their early childhood development services for children under age 6 (Government of Canada Federal, 2004). The provincial and territorial governments, excluding Quebec province, which manages its own social affairs, are required to focus on four national action areas. Each government has different approaches and programs, but all use a common reporting measure to promote comparison. The action areas are:

- Promote healthy pregnancy, birth, and infancy
- Improve parenting and family supports
- Strengthen early childhood development, learning, and care
- Strengthen community supports (Government of Canada Federal, 2004)

Early childhood education services consist of child care during parental work hours and preschool programs that teach and socially prepare children for school. Both services are publicly subsidized and provide preference to children from low-income families and those with developmental delays or other special needs (Kamerman, 2000). Canada also has a Universal Child Care Plan (the Plan) and Universal Child Care Benefit, which allows parents the choice of the most appropriate type of child care and provides financial resources for parents regardless of their location, circumstances, or preferences (Government of Canada, 2009).

Canada has a nationally known, community-based early intervention effort, the Better Beginnings Better Futures project, which was designed to reduce emotional and behavioral problems in young children. The model relies on significant parent and community participation and uses strategies chosen by the beneficiaries (Peters, 2004). Evaluations of the program have shown decreases in social and emotional problems, improved health outcomes, increased preventive health care use, and increases in linking young children with early intervention and other services (Peters, 2000).

Russia

Background, Demographics, and Prevalence

The Russian Federation spans the largest area of any country. As of 2009, its population is an estimated 140,041,247, with 14.8 percent under the age of 15 (United States Central Intelligence Agency, 2009d). Poor economic conditions are widespread in Russia, especially in rural areas. According to UNICEF statistics, Russia has one of the highest infant mortality rates (under age 1) in Eastern Europe at 13 per 1,000 live births in 2007 (UNICEF, 2009).

There are special considerations in Russia with regard to vulnerable children. The first is the number of children living in state-run institutions and on the streets. Although labeled as orphans, many of these children have been abandoned by their parents or live on the streets due to domestic abuse. USAID reports that in 2007, there were almost 732,000 children in orphanages, and *2 million to 4 million* street or neglected ("unsupervised") children in Russia (Telyukov & Paterson, 2009).

The second special consideration is the high number of children with disabilities. UNICEF reports that 2.5 percent of Russian children are registered as having a disability with the health and social security authorities. There are over 62,000 children with disabilities in Russian state institutions as of 2002. However, many institutionalized children with disabilities are not registered with the social security administration. In actuality, UNICEF estimates that there were 174,432 children with disabilities in Russian institutions in 2002 (UNICEF, 2005).

Key Early Intervention Issues

The national framework for special education was conceived in Russia when the first schools for children with vision and hearing disorders were founded by Alexander I in 1806. After the 1917 revolution, church and state separated, and any kind of charity was forbidden. As a result, all special education schools and shelters for people with disabilities, which were usually church-based, lost financial and political support (Malofeev, 1996, 2000).

At that time, Russia was experiencing a unique and drastic change in its political and economic systems, ideology, values, and cultural norms, along with deep economic crisis and civil war. The new government took responsibility to educate children with developmental disorders.

The conditions on which the system of special education in the Soviet Russia was being formed were tough: there was no education-for-all legislation and no Individuals with Disabilities Education Act, no possibility to interact with parents and civil movements, and no philanthropy. The only financial resource was the government (Malofeev, 2000).

During the late 1920s and early 1930s, the need for a special education system for people with hearing, vision, and mental disabilities was recognized. This policy was the "General Compulsory Education Act" created by a resolution passed on July 25, 1930. However, this document applied only to public schools; therefore, special education schools were required to follow common school standards that were applied to all children regardless of their abilities. Those with mental and physical disabilities were considered "uneducable" and excluded from public schools. Special boarding schools without any education programs were founded for these children.

During the 1950s–1990s, a system was established that included eight types of special education schools and 15 types of special education programs. Nevertheless, in reality, not more than 3 percent of all schoolchildren had the ability to study there. In addition, special education schools and properly trained teachers were spread unevenly throughout the country.

When the Soviet Union collapsed, the country and its people once again faced fundamental changes in culture, economics, and society. In 1991, the Russian Federation proclaimed itself a democratic country and ratified the CRC, the Convention of the Rights of Persons with Disabilities, and the Rights of Mentally Retarded Persons. Upon ratification, attitudes toward people with disabilities were expected to change. However, the system of care and education for children with special needs continued to lack the integration of care and education, identification of children at risk, and early intervention programs. A great number of children with developmental disabilities were sent to orphanages and later were raised in boarding schools.

By the time the first early intervention program was established in Russia, the national demographics, health conditions and quality of life of children had reached dire states. According to data in the Governmental Report, "On Childhood Conditions in the Russian Federation" (1994), there was a decrease in the birthrate from 17.2 to 9.4 per 1,000 inhabitants in Russia from 1987 to 1993; an increase in the morbidity of neonates (173.7 babies per 1,000 live births in 1991 as compared to 82.4 in 1980); and an increased infant mortality rate.

Until recently, Russian infant facilities in general, and particularly those for at-risk babies, provided medical assistance but no educational, psychological, or social-work supports. Therefore, when left in the family, high-risk children had no access to medical assistance, and families of babies with special needs had virtually no choice between a segregated institution and keeping the child at home. High-risk babies were often taken away from the family and placed in special, medically oriented institutions. Infant facilities lacked screening and assessment techniques for infants' development. In addition, limited current research on infant development was available for parents or professionals. Until recently, the universities and pedagogical institutes have focused on training specialists to work with children over the age of 3. There were no preservice programs for teachers (including special education) or psychologists for children in early childhood, and no professional training in such specialties as motor development or organizing the settings for very young children (physical and occupational therapy; Muhamedrahimov, 2000).

National Policies and Programs

Since 1991, the government of the Russian Federation passed more than 300 regulatory acts protecting the rights of children with disabilities. Legislative possibilities for formulating the Early Intervention Act were created. However, the project itself is in the process of discussion, and modifications are being made according to early intervention and inclusive education practices since 1992. Russia is one of the few developed countries that have not yet adopted a nondiscrimination law that guarantees citizens with disabilities the right to special education (extract from a letter to the Government of Russia from the Education Academy, 2007). On April 24, 2006, in the course of Parliament proceedings, three obstacles were outlined: (1) no common system of early diagnosis or child and family psychological follow-up, (2) difficulties in creating proper conditions for the development of early intervention programs in state institutions, and (3) teachers were not trained properly and systematically to work in this field (Policy Brief of the Russian Academy of Education to the Government of the Russian Federation, 2007). In 2006, the right to develop policies in the field of early intervention and the creation of necessary conditions for them was legalized (122 Federal Law, 22.08.2004) and was provided to the local and regional governments. Depending on the social and economic status of the region, the social politics, and the number of specialists available, several key trends exist (Razenkova, 2009):

1. Integrating professional training initiatives into regional laws and distribution of evidence-based early intervention models. This trend has existed in St. Petersburg since 1991.
2. Initiatives to legally require early intervention programs stem from the regional government. During this time, various models of serving children and their parents are being created (Moscow, Samara region, Krasnoyarsk region). In these cases, programs are opened as branches of existing state institutions of the education, health, and social defense systems.
3. The development of separate non-state initiatives serving children with special needs and their parents is essentially financed by international grants. Usually, non-state initiatives are a cooperation of the nongovernmental organization (NGO) and the government institutions (Downside Up, the charity fund, Moscow; The National Foundation for the Prevention of Cruelty to Children [NFPCC], Moscow).

In November 2009, the Russian government, in cooperation with UNICEF Russia, launched a series of Children's Rights public service announcements (PSAs). These PSAs were broadcast via video, billboards, and magazines and were scheduled to run through March 1, 2010, in commemoration of the 20th anniversary of the Convention of the Rights of the Child (UNICEF, 2009). The announcements emphasize societal responsibility to all children, especially children at risk.

China

Background and Demographics

The People's Republic of China (PRC) is a vast and diverse country culturally, economically, and geographically, which is influenced by both Eastern and Western traditions. Many ethnic groups comprise its population of about 1.3 billion (United States Central Intelligence Agency, 2009c). The country is divided into 22 provinces, 5 autonomous areas, 4 municipalities, and a special administrative region. National reforms since the late 1970s have improved the standard of living throughout PRC, but disparities between regions are great. The coastal areas and eastern provinces are more populated and developed than the eastern and rural areas (Tsai-Hsing, McCabe, & Bao-Jen, 2003). Many children live in rural and underresourced communities (McLoughlin, Zhou, & Clark, 2005).

Historically in PRC, children with disabilities were viewed as society's responsibility and were accorded public sympathy, yet these children rarely received education outside of the home until the first schools for the blind and deaf were built by Western missionaries in the late 1800s (Chen, 1996). Prior to their creation, cultural norms and government policies often excluded children with disabilities from public education. In the last 60 years, dramatic and fundamental economic, social, and cultural changes occurred in PRC that affected the availability of services for children with a range of abilities. Social, political, and economic reforms in the late 1970s resulted in a growing acceptance of differences of ability, which led to changes in the education system that offered more support for children with special needs (McCabe, 2003).

Key Early Intervention Issues/Prevalence

The contemporary concept of disability is defined in the 1987 National Survey on the Status of Disability (NSSD). A number of factors make accurate estimation of prevalence of childhood disability difficult. PRC lacks well-designed, large-scale studies and an organized collection of national statistics on early childhood disabilities. There is no standard measure of child development in PRC, and the data from Western tools that have been adapted to the local culture are not always interpreted correctly, and few professionals are trained to administer these tests (McLoughlin et al., 2005). Many children with disabilities are delayed in receiving diagnosis and treatment due to the cultural perception that a medical professional should identify a disability rather than a caregiver or educator (McLoughlin et al., 2005).

The prevalence of disabilities in children birth to 4 years is 2.9 percent, and the most common disabilities are hearing impairment, intellectual disability, and physical impairment (Asia-Pacific Development Center on Disability, 2002). The NSSD estimated there were 2.46 million special needs children under age 6 (Epstein, 1992; Gargiulo, 1996; Odom, 2003; Tsai-Hsing et al., 2003). Preliminary findings of the second National Survey (2006–2007) show the proportion of disabled persons to the total population has increased since 1987 (China Disabled Persons' Federation, 2006). A 2002 survey estimated that 4.3 million people live with disabilities in PRC. Its immense population makes PRC the country with the most individuals with special needs. Stratford and Ng (2000) estimate that a child with a disability is born in PRC every 40 seconds, or about 2,000 births per day. This is striking, considering the United States Census Bureau estimates that one child—with or without a disability—is born every seven seconds the United States.

A reported 62.5 percent of the country's children with special needs receive education (Asia-Pacific Development Center on Disability, 2002). About 15 percent of those students attended special education schools, 8 percent attended specialized classes, and over 77 percent were educated in regular classes. However, many children with special needs did not attend any school due to a lack of sufficient school placements and teachers, classrooms, and trained teachers (McCabe, 2003).

National Early Intervention Policies and Programs

The value placed on education by Chinese culture and the push for compulsory education has led to policies that increase access to appropriate early education for children with special needs. The Compulsory Education Act of 1986 required all levels of government to provide nine years of education to all children in general or specialized schools or classes (Chen, 1996; Disability Rights Education and Defense Fund, Seventh National People's Congress, 1986).

The 1990 Law of the People's Republic of China on the Basic Protection of Disabled Persons was the first legislation to encourage special education programs in early childhood in addition to elementary schools (Disability Rights Education and Defense Fund, Seventh National People's Congress, 1990). Article 25 states that preschools and primary and junior high schools must accept students with disabilities who are "able to adapt themselves to life there." For children who do require specialized services or classrooms, Article 26 adds that preschools and schools must provide for those children's needs through schools dedicated to children with disabilities or specialized classrooms attached to general education schools or welfare institutions (Disability Rights Education and Defense Fund, 1990).

The Compulsory Education Law (1986) led to better integration of children with special needs into general education classrooms. Often, basic education is achieved in inclusive classrooms to due to practical necessity. The concept of inclusion is called *Suiban Jinudo*, and initially resulted from the inability of many schools in resource-constrained or rural areas to build special schools. Thus, these villages integrated all children into general education classrooms. However, few teachers are trained in special needs instruction techniques, and there is little oversight of the implementation of *Suiban Jiudu* in schools (Pang, 2006).

Many localities have begun the integration in preschool (at age 3 1/2), believing earlier integration will assist primary schools to better educate all children with minimal modifications necessary (McCabe, 2003; Pang, 2006). To integrate at the preschool level, a variety of approaches have been used, including: completely integrated class-rooms; integrated classrooms that use instructional modifications or segregate children for some activities; and others that have developed counterpart arrangements between general education schools and those with special education programs (McCabe, 2003).

Children's rights were extended into early childhood through the Law on the Basic Protection for the Disabled and the Regulations on Education for Persons with Disabilities (1994), which identified national policy goals to develop and improve services for individuals with special needs and prioritized the development of early interven-tion programs (Chen, 1996). Together, these policies led to an increase in the number of children with special needs attending preschools (Pang, 2006; McCabe, 2003). Early intervention services are delivered in a variety of ways, including public or private schools, rehabilitation centers, and other organizations. Currently, many services are deliv-ered in early intervention classes within special education schools, but more and more schools are integrating general education and spe-cial needs students (Tsai-Hsing et al., 2003; McLoughlin et al., 2005).

PRC uses some of the early intervention models developed in the United States and other Western countries, such as the Head Start model, to intervene on behalf of young children with disabilities and those who are at risk (Tsai-Hsing et al., 2003). However, economic and material resources can be scarce, especially in rural areas that often lack trained professionals and interdisciplinary agencies to con-duct interventions (Tsai-Hsing et al., 2003). However, since the 1980s, PRC has made substantial progress toward developing early interven-tion and special education programs in rural and resource-constrained areas (Deng, 2004; Tsai-Hsing et al., 2003). Since then, more commun-ities have begun to offer preschool programs for children with special needs, and many children with mild to moderate disabilities were included in general preschool classes. While the number of early child-hood intervention and special education services is growing, there is much work to be done to increase the capacity and quality of services (Odom, 2003; Tsai-Hsing et al., 2003; Zhao, Guo, & Zhou, 1997).

Parents have played an important role in improving early intervention and special education services in PRC, but on the whole, parents and providers could improve their partnership. Parents have lobbied effectively for the creation of community schools for children with disabilities, yet special education teachers often struggle to establish relationships with some parents due to the parental perception that teachers are the authorities whose expertise should be respected. Some parents also feel shame at having a child with a disability and do not draw attention to it (McCabe, 2003). As in other countries, many Chinese households have two working parents or face economic hardship, making parental involvement challenging (Tsai-Hsing et al., 2003). Some programs also offer education and support for parents of children with special needs.

PRC's policy of limiting the majority of couples to having only one child (known as the "One Child Policy") has influenced some parents' relationships with their children. When a firstborn child has a disability, parents may apply for permission to have a second child. Although some families have abandoned a child born with disabilities, many others have been able to devote significant time, attention, and resources to their child with special needs. In many families, four grandparents and two parents are all available to offer one child a wealth of care and support (Tsai-Hsing et al., 2003).

New Zealand

Background and Demographics

New Zealand is a small but growing agricultural country with a population of 4,280,000 and a beautiful and diverse terrain. The majority of the population is descended from Europeans, Maori, Asian, and other Polynesian Pacific heritages. Education is compulsory from ages 6 to 16. The country enjoys a low infant mortality rate and high life expectancy. New Zealand is led by a prime minister and is an independent member of the Commonwealth of Nations, a group of countries that were formerly British colonies (New Zealand Statistics, 2006).

Incidence and Prevalence

The 2006 census reports the population birth to age 4 was approximately 286,000, with an estimated 5.2 percent prevalence of all disability in this group. About four-fifths of these children receive supportive services (New Zealand Statistics, 2006; Dalziel, 2001). The most common types of disability are chronic conditions and diseases that existed at birth, which affect 4 percent of children, and psychiatric or psychological disorders, affecting 2 percent. An estimated 5 percent of children required special educational considerations due to a chronic health problem, or a learning or developmental disorder. Data are also kept on other common disability types such as speech, sight, hearing, and intellectual disorders. Fifty-two percent of children had a single disability, while 48 percent had multiple disabilities. Eighty-six percent of these children require "low" (41%) to "medium" (45%) level supports (Bascand, 2006).

The New Zealand Disability Strategy

The New Zealand Disability Strategy (the Strategy) outlines steps to achieve an inclusive society that supports full participation of all people with any type of disability. The Strategy was developed by the Ministry of Health in consultation with people living with disabilities, their families, and a group of organizations working on disability-related issues. A committee of experts on disability, the Sector Reference Group, was established by the minister for disability to advise the content and development of the strategy. This group and the Ministry of Health first drafted and produced a discussion document, which was released and debated at 68 public meetings throughout New Zealand. Over 700 people responded, including individuals with disabilities, their families, extended familial networks, service providers, and advocates for people with disabilities. The Sector Reference Group analyzed the findings and presented their recommendations to the minister for disability issues. The revised draft later became the Strategy, launched on April 30, 2001.

In 15 objectives and 113 actions, the Strategy outlines objectives covering all aspects of life including education; human and legal rights; lifestyle choices; access to information; inclusion of minority groups; special attention to children, youth, and women; and the value of families and other sources of support (New Zealand Office of Disability Issues, 2009). The scope of the Strategy goes beyond providing high-quality support services, although that is an integral component. The developers of the Strategy recognize that most of the barriers encountered by individuals with disabilities are associated with public ignorance or stigmas, violations of human rights, and unequal access to educational and employment opportunities. The vision proposed in the Strategy is a society that places high value on the lives of people with disabilities and strives to enhance their participation (New Zealand Office of Disability Issues, 2009).

To this end, the Strategy requires government agencies to consider the implications of their decision making on people with disabilities. The document is organized around five key themes: upholding citizenship, building government capacity, improving support services, promoting participation in all areas of life, and addressing diversity of need (Dalziel, 2001). Fifteen objectives that embody a rights-based approach to disability are enumerated in the Strategy; several directly affect children with special needs (New Zealand Office of Disability Issues, 2008a).

The first step of implementation focused on government agencies incorporating the Strategy objectives in their services, funding, and policy development. The Office of Disability Issues also works with public agencies to reduce stigma surrounding people with disabilities. Local authorities have the responsibility to improve access to community resources. The Strategy operates across sectors and complements other national policies such as the New Zealand Health Strategy (New Zealand Office of Disability Issues, 2009). Progress in implementation is monitored through required reports submitted by all government agencies. The minister for disability issues oversees progress and reports yearly to Parliament on progress and challenges. The Office for Disability is responsible for promoting the Strategy and monitoring implementation. Nongovernmental organizations, a nonprofit organization with an international focus, are invited to participate as well (New Zealand Office of Disability Issues, 2008b).

Some objectives of the Strategy are pertinent to children. Objective 3 of the Strategy focuses on eight actions designed to ensure a quality education. The action steps promote the right of all persons to education, use of communication techniques to enhance learning, trained and knowledgeable instructors who are sensitive to the needs of disabled students, equitable access to resources, the right to appropriate and effective inclusive education, access to peer interaction among students with disabilities, school accountability, and development of higher education options for students with disabilities (Dalziel, 2001). In New Zealand, inclusive education means the right of every student to learn and fully participate in an integrated classroom with other children his or her age (Ballard, 1996).

Objective 13 outlines 10 action steps to enable children and youth to lead full and active lives. These actions embody the values of early intervention in New Zealand. Action 1 notes the importance of interdisciplinary coordination, collaboration, and leadership among agencies working with children, youth, and families, which are necessary to provide appropriate services that recognize the particular needs of children with disabilities. Other action steps include conducting public education and antidiscrimination campaigns, developing family-focused support services, including the input of disabled people in policy and program formulation, and taking other steps to promote independent living and greater control in the lives of persons with disabilities (Dalziel, 2001).

In addition to the Strategy, the New Zealand Public Health and Disability Act 2000 (NZPHD Act) guides the organization and funding of health and disability services in New Zealand. Its goals include improving health outcomes, reducing health disparities, disseminating information, fully including people with disabilities, and providing opportunity for all New Zealanders to provide input into public health and disability services (New Zealand Ministry of Health, 2000).

Brazil

Background and Demographics

At over three million square miles, Brazil is the world's fifth-largest country by geography, comprising almost half of the South American continent. It is a federal republic, which means the country is led by a national government and constitution, with 26 self-governing states, 1 federal district, and more than 5,500 local municipalities. The 2000 census shows a population over 170 million. About 23 million children, or 13.5 percent of the population, are preschool aged (Freitas, Shelton, & Tudge, 2008). The census estimates 14.5 percent of the population live with a disability (Mont, 2007).

Brazil's people are experiencing a major shift in age and demographics and a rapidly declining fertility rate. Poverty affects all urban areas, especially those in the northeast region, and nonwhite individuals and those living in rural areas experience higher rates of poverty (Lumpkin & Aranha, 2003). Brazil is reported to have the most unequal distribution of wealth among its citizens of any county in the world, resulting in dramatic imbalances in the ability to access education and social services (Lumpkin & Aranha, 2003; Celia, 2004).

In 1988, Brazil ended military rule, adopted a constitution, and began national decentralization in which more authority and responsibility shifted from the national to local governments. Many municipalities struggle to fill their new responsibilities of providing health and human services; however, the country is making an effort to build the capacity of local governments. Article 227 of the national constitution ensures that the human rights of all children shall be upheld and protected by families, society, and the government at all levels. The adoption of the new constitution coincided with the Convention on the Rights of the Child and the passing of two seminal laws in 1990 (Statute of the Child and Adolescent and the Lei Organica da Suade) to form an era of recognition and support for child rights (Lumpkin & Aranha, 2003).

Brazil is part of a regional movement in Latin America and the Caribbean (LAC) to coordinate the efforts to protect child rights and guarantee their healthy development and active participation in society. Marked improvements have occurred since the 1990s, yet the progress among countries varies widely. Often the neglected areas or those last addressed by reform are services for the youngest children and children at risk for or with disabilities.

Brazil's education system is decentralized, with clear domains drawn among levels of government. Local municipalities are responsible for providing and guaranteeing access to early childhood development services, such as child care, preschool, and kindergarten. Increasingly, municipalities are also responsible for primary education, formerly shared between state and local authorities. Secondary education is provided by states, while the federal government devises education standards and attempts to reduce educational disparities through equalizing material and funding distribution (Lumpkin & Aranha, 2003). The majority of children receive a free public education. Primary education is guaranteed for all, and special education has shifted toward an inclusive model. In 1998, about 87 percent of children with disabilities received education services in special schools. By 2000, 79 percent attended special schools and 21 percent attended inclusive schools (Lumpkin & Aranha, 2003). Education at all ages has increased, including the rate of preschool enrollment (Celia, 2004). Because Brazil is a large, populous, and diverse country, it is challenging to design and implement public policies that meet the needs of all children while implementing quality standards and maintaining respect for cultural, ethnic, and regional diversity (Freitas et al., 2008).

Key Early Intervention Issues and Prevalence

Brazil's new constitution recognized children's and their families' rights from birth. The 1991 Statute of the Child and Adolescent (often referred to as the Children's Constitution) also declared children's rights as citizens who are entitled to protection and free education. Public Law on the Rights and Basis of Education (Public Law), created in 1996, integrated education from birth to age 6 into the public education system. The Public Law recognized early childhood as the foundation of basic education; supported the coordination of school, community, and family-based socialization efforts; and established a minimum standard of early childhood development knowledge for teachers of young children. In 2004, an estimated 1.3 million children (10%) from birth to age 3 attended day care, and another 5.6 million (56%) aged 4 to 6 attended preschool. The majority of these programs are located in urban areas, reflecting the 86 percent of the population that lives there (United States Central Intelligence Agency, 2009a), but resulting in unequal distribution of early childhood education (Freitas et al., 2008). The constitution also gave legal legitimacy to the social norm that parents and extended families are considered the first providers of care and support to children (Lumpkin & Aranha, 2003).

National Early Intervention Policies and National-Level Programs

Brazil has taken a unique approach to early intervention while increasing primary school enrollment and reducing child labor rates. Guided by the Federal Secretariat of Social Assistance (SEAS), state and municipal governments collaborate on numerous programs designed to enhance family support and capacity and increase primary education through financial incentives based on school attendance. These early intervention programs exist for children with disabilities and children at risk. SEAS's main objectives are to coordinate services and provide all levels of government and nongovernmental agencies with technical and financial support that promotes protective measures and social inclusion. SEAS partners with other funding agencies to enhance institutional capacity at child care centers, and community-based primary health care initiatives targeting pregnant women and children under age 6 are supported and prioritized at all levels of government. There, identification of children with special needs is frequently done through community health outreach workers and volunteers (Lumpkin & Aranha, 2003).

Legally, all children have the right to education from birth, resulting in a large percentage of children enrolled in early childhood education programs (Freitas et al., 2008). The inclusion model is becoming more common in primary school, but organized early intervention programs are few. Many parents are not informed of their child's rights and are unable or unwilling to dedicate the necessary time to fight for those rights. Most groups working on behalf of children with disabilities focus on a few key issues, resulting in fragmentation among early intervention and childhood disability efforts (Freitas et al., 2008).

A lack of coordination among the health, education, and social services sectors hampers early childhood initiatives, family support services, and early intervention efforts. Add to that redundancy of service and conflict among public agencies, nongovernmental organizations, and parent-led groups. While progress to include individuals with disabilities into the policy process has been made, many families still lack knowledge of, and access to, preventive and early intervention services (Lumpkin & Aranha, 2003).

South Africa

Background and Demographics

South Africa, population 49 million, is a middle-income country that has well-developed business, legal, and communications sectors; is rich in natural resources; and is a strong player in the global market. The population is comprised of four self-classified groups: black African, colored, Indian or Asian, and white. Among these groups, significant disparities in living conditions, opportunity, and social circumstances persist. Poverty, unemployment, and political and social marginalization are persistent effects of South Africa's history of legal racial segregation and discrimination that perpetuate disparities in many aspects of life, including early childhood services (United States Central Intelligence Agency, 2009e). Persons with disabilities are more likely to experience poverty, social isolation, and unemployment during all phases of life, and great disparities in access to and use of social services exist (McClain et al., 1997).

South Africa's policy objectives regarding disability issues include raising awareness, decreasing discrimination, and valuing diversity among citizens. Its movement toward a "social model" values the participation of individuals with disabilities and proposes increased inclusion in decision-making processes (McClain et al., 1997). Insufficient coordination exists among government agencies to properly implement preventive measures, early identification, or early intervention for children. Public awareness and political support is increasing, but there is an ongoing failure to implement policies created to support them (Saloojee, Phohole, Saloojee, & Ijsselmuiden, 2006).

Key EI issues and Prevalence

The most commonly cited prevalence estimates of motor, sensory, and intellectual impairments in children birth to age 9 are 5.2 to 6.4 percent (Anderson, 1991; Case, 1999; Christianson, et al. 2002; Corneljie, 1991; Couper, 2002, as cited in Saloojee et al., 2006), but some estimates put the prevalence rate of moderate-to-severe impairments as high as 12 percent (McClain et al., 1997). The President's Integrated Disability Strategy (the Strategy) acknowledges a lack of reliable information on the prevalence and type of disabilities experienced by South African children. Data gathering on disability is hindered by multiple definitions of disability, lack of common data-gathering techniques, discrimination, poor infrastructure, and periodic violence that interrupts data collection and service provision (McClain et al., 1997).

Historically, disability has been framed as a medical rather than a social issue, resulting in social isolation and a lack of national statistics on disability. Reflecting changing global attitudes, South Africa is working to reframe its cultural and social perceptions of disability to create a more inclusive environment. One key aspect of this change is participation of persons with special needs in policy development (McClain et al., 1997). Secondly, there has been a professional ideological shift toward understanding the context in which children develop, considering parent-child interactions, building collaborations between families and professionals, and developing multi-sector responses to early childhood issues (Eloff, 2006).

Early childhood intervention services face a number of challenges including poverty, high unemployment, low literacy rates, and urgent public health concerns such as HIV/AIDS. There are also a large number of young children in the population, yet few early childhood services for them. The national government has recently made a commitment to early childhood education that will require a national-level social reconstruction that addresses poverty and disparities in access to health care and education (Eloff, 2006). To improve access to services, professionals must also understand family perceptions of disability. Often, families take a fatalistic view of any type of impairment a child may be born with or develop in course of life, a belief that may decrease their likelihood to seek intervention. Families and professionals must partner to achieve the best outcomes, and professionals must have culturally specific knowledge and techniques.

National Policies and Programs

In South Africa, "educare" is the term commonly used by nongovernmental organizations to refer to services for young children. It conveys that there is no formal line between education and caregiving services, yet government agencies divide education and care services between different departments and funding streams, resulting in a lack of coordination and consistency between communities and among the levels of government. "Day care" is controlled by the Department of Health, but "preschool education" falls under Department of Education. Each department operates independently (Liddell & Kemp, 1995).

The quality of ECD services varies greatly throughout the country. Children under age 5 are served through both public and independent ECD programs. Most public programs are funded by the provincial Department of Education and provide pre-primary schools for children aged 3 to 5. Independent programs offer a wider variety of services and are funded through a combination of fees, fund-raising, and limited governmental support. Independent services are usually provided in community-based sites or independent pre-primary schools. After a review of nearly 22,000 ECD sites, the Ministry of Education estimates 49 percent are community-based, 34 percent are home-based, and 17 percent are school-based (Asmal, 2001a).

One of the challenges facing postapartheid South Africa is overcoming the history of discrimination and realizing the constitutional value of equity provided to all learners. Historically, services for children were segregated based on race and special need (Walton, Nel, Hugo, & Muller, 2009). Since 2004, all individuals with disabilities were also entitled to free health services as well as basic education guaranteed by the constitution. The families of children with special needs may also receive a "care dependency grant" of about $110 USD (Saloojee et al., 2006, page 231). The Office on the Status of Disabled Persons in the Office of the Deputy President works with state departments and nongovernmental organizations to promote, create, and maintain an environment that encourages acceptance of and equal participation by individuals with special needs (McClain et al., 1997). The country's Integrated Disability Strategy White Paper asserts South Africa will follow the precedent set in the United Nations Standard Rules for the Equalization of Opportunities for Persons with Disabilities and the World Program of Action Concerning Disabled Persons, thereby following a rights-based philosophy (McClain et al., 1997).

This approach requires major changes in many of South Africa's education sites. Historically, children were classified and segregated into special schools or rooms according to their ability. Many schools, especially those in rural areas, were neither able nor willing to accommodate special needs children. As of the late 1990s, an estimated 70 percent of children with special needs did not attend school. Government publications since then have proposed to integrate all children in both traditional and dedicated service centers (McClain et al., 1997). The public education sector is currently enacting a 20-year plan to promote inclusion and full participation of children with special needs into general education schools (Saloojee et al., 2006), and also plans to improve out-of-classroom opportunities that promote life skills development, independent living, and workforce training (McClain et al., 1997).

Early intervention services in South Africa are influenced by a number of postapartheid national policies. In 1998, the Department of Education reviewed national health, education, and social welfare policies and programs that impact early childhood development and concluded that policies and programs had been adopted at all levels of government. Some of the major policies are mentioned below.

The Child Care Act 74 (1983) guided the first early childhood development policies. The Early Childhood Development White Paper from the Department of Education (2001) updated the country's early childhood development philosophy and is the guiding document for implementation of early childhood programs (UNESCO, 2006). It established the National Early Childhood Program, largely focused on 4- to 5-year olds transitioning into school. The program and policy goals set in this document and applicable to children birth to age 5 include a national curriculum, professional development and career-track planning programs for providers, an accreditation program for providers, and a national information and advocacy outreach program for parents and communities (UNESCO, 2006). The White Paper identifies a need to develop services and programs for children under age 4 with special education needs, among other "special populations" in need of more focused attention and service provision at the local, state, and national levels (Asmal, 2001a).

In 1997, the Integrated National Disability Strategy (the Strategy) was published, which frames inclusive education as the foundation on which to build an integrated society. The Strategy proposes that all early childhood education be provided in an environment that acknowledges, accepts, and values diversity. Furthermore, to meet the country's goal of forming an integrated society, education must be equally accessible to all children regardless of the nature of their needs. If the existing school system cannot appropriately serve a child with special needs, the child should have access to a school that can. Finally, parents' rights and preferences for their children should be given consideration. The Strategy proposes to have children with special needs access education services earlier, and it targets vulnerable populations, such as black African children, girls, very young children, those with multiple disabilities, and those living in rural areas (McClain et al., 1997).

Also in 1997, the report *Quality Education for All: Overcoming Barriers to Learning and Development* was published. This document recommended increased focus on early identification, assessment, and intervention for children with special education needs. Another document, the *Inter-Ministerial Committee on Young People at Risk*, made policy recommendations for increased focus on prevention, building child resilience, and early intervention (Asmal, 2001a).

Despite these policies, approximately 82 percent of early childhood programs designed for children up to age 5 serve only 3- to 5-year olds. Services for children under age 3 are lacking, despite acknowledgement from the Ministry of Education that this is the most crucial time of child development (Asmal, 2001a). Early childhood development programs are viewed as a form of investment in human and economic development for the country; however, the primary responsibility for the care of children rests with families. The Early Childhood Development strategic plan focuses on delivering inclusive and appropriate services, prioritizes the development of a national early childhood curriculum, advancing professional development for teachers and caregivers, and improving the physical conditions in schools and child care centers (Asmal, 2001b).

In 2008, the Parliament enacted the Children's Act to reflect the contemporary views of children's rights that appear in the constitution and the CRC. This act protects the most vulnerable groups of children and encourages the creation of a national policy model for children's social development. The legislation provides families with policy and

Key Aspects of Policies	Brazil	Canada	China	New Zealand	Russia	South Africa
The Convention on the Rights of the Child (1989)						
Nondiscrimination	1988 Constitution	1985 Human Rights Act	1982 Constitution	The NZ Disability Strategy	1993 Constitution	1996 Constitution
Devotion to the best interests of the child	91 Children's Constitution	2000 ECD Communique		1989 Children, Young Persons & Families Act		2001 ECD White Paper
All children have the right to life, survival, and development	1988 Constitution	2000 ECD Communique	1991 L.P.M.~	1989 Children, Young Persons & Families Act	1995 Family Code	1996 Constitution
Respect for the views of the child	91 Children's Constitution			1989 Children, Young Persons & Families Act		1992 Children's Charter of S.A.
All children and families must be informed of, and receive, appropriate care and services	Programa Bolsa Familia	2000 ECD Communique		1989 Children, Young Persons & Families Act		2005 Children's Act
There should be no financial barriers to services	Programa Bolsa Familia	2006 Univ. Child Care Plan		1989 Children, Young Persons & Families Act	1993 Constitution	1992 Children's Charter of S.A.
Focuses on the unique needs and vulnerabilities of children under age 18	91 Children's Constitution		1991 L.P.M.~	1989 Children, Young Persons & Families Act	2002 Pres. Order for I.C.A.M.***	1996 Constitution
All countries should recognize a child's right to an adequate standard of living for physical, mental, spiritual, moral and social development	91 Children's Constitution	2000 ECD Communique	1991 L.P.M.~	1989 Children, Young Persons & Families Act		1996 Constitution
Universal Declaration of Human Rights (1948)						
Childhood is recognized as a unique time deserving of special care, assistance, and protection	91 Children's Constitution		1991 L.P.M.~	1989 Children, Young Persons & Families Act	1993 Constitution	1992 Children's Charter of S.A.
Established the essential worth of human beings, giving political support to all people of all countries, ethnicities, genders, religions, and socio-economic backgrounds	91 Children's Constitution	1985 Human Rights Act	1982 Constitution	1989 Children, Young Persons & Families Act	1993 Constitution	1996 Constitution
Declaration on the Rights of Disabled Persons (1975)						
All children should receive services tailored to their needs	91 Children's Constitution		1990 BPDP Law*	The NZ Disability Strategy	1995 Law on S.P.P.D.**	2001 ECD White Paper
Children with special needs have a right to appropriate treatments	91 Children's Constitution	Universal Healthcare	1990 BPDP Law*	The NZ Disability Strategy	1995 Law on S.P.P.D.**	1997 INDS~~
Children with special needs have a right to environments and living conditions that are as appropriate and equivalent as possible to those of their contemporaries	91 Children's Constitution		1990 BPDP Law*	The NZ Disability Strategy	1995 Law on S.P.P.D.**	2001 ECD White Paper
Integration of mixed-ability individuals		1985 Human Rights Act	1986 Compulsory Edu. Act	The NZ Disability Strategy	1995 Law on S.P.P.D.**	
Jomtien Declaration (1990)						
Declares that learning begins at birth	1996 Public Law	2000 ECD Communique		Pathways to the Future		2001 ECD White Paper
Recognizes early childhood care and education as an integral part of basic education	1996 Public Law	2000 ECD Communique	1989 Kindergarten regulations	Pathways to the Future	1993 Constitution	2001 ECD White Paper
Early childhood care and education should be provided in multiple settings	1996 Public Law	2006 Univ. Child Care Plan		Pathways to the Future		2001 ECD White Paper
All children have the right to educational opportunities such as literacy, numeracy, problem solving, and life skill development	1988 Constitution	2006 Univ. Child Care Plan	1986 Compulsory Edu. Act	The NZ Disability Strategy		1997 INDS~~
Basic education is the right of all children, regardless of situation or ability	1988 Constitution	2006 Univ. Child Care Plan	1986 Compulsory Edu. Act	The NZ Disability Strategy	1993 Constitution	1997 INDS~~
The Standard Rules on Equalization Opportunities for Persons with Disabilities (1993)						
State should provide multidisciplinary professional teams for early detection, assessment, and treatment of disabilities	91 Children's Constitution	2000 ECD Communique	1990 BPDP Law*	The NZ Disability Strategy	1995 Law on S.P.P.D.**	1997 INDS~~
Rehabilitation should be provided in appropriate ways that maximize equal participation in society	91 Children's Constitution	2000 ECD Communique	1990 BPDP Law*	The NZ Disability Strategy	1995 Law on S.P.P.D.**	1997 INDS~~
Recognizes that very young children need special consideration	91 Children's Constitution	2000 ECD Communique	1990 BPDP Law*	The NZ Disability Strategy		1997 INDS~~
Promotes inclusive, culturally-sensitive, and appropriate education for all children	2001 Nat'l. Edu. Plan	2000 ECD Communique	1986 Compulsory Edu. Act	The NZ Disability Strategy	1995 Law on S.P.P.D.**	2001 Special Needs Edu. White Paper
Salamanca Statement (1994)						
Promotes inclusion and integrated schools	2001 Nat'l. Edu.Plan	Provincial Governments**		The NZ Disability Strategy	1995 Law on S.P.P.D.**	2001 Special Needs Edu. White Paper
Communities should embrace differences in ability	2001 Nat'l. Edu.Plan	1985 Human Rights Act	1990 BPDP Law*	The NZ Disability Strategy	1995 Law on S.P.P.D.**	2001 Special Needs Edu. White Paper
Respond to individuals' unique needs	2001 Nat'l. Edu.Plan	1985 Human Rights Act	1990 BPDP Law*	The NZ Disability Strategy	1995 Law on S.P.P.D.**	1997 INDS~~
Dakar Framework for Action (2000)						
All children have a right to free and compulsory education regardless of resources of the home country	2001 Nat'l. Edu.Plan (to age 14)	Provincial Governments**	1986 Compulsory Edu. Act	The NZ Disability Strategy	1993 Constitution	1992 Children's Charter of S.A.
Promotes expansion and improvement of early childhood care and education for all children	2001 Nat'l. Edu.Plan	2000 ECD Communique	1994 Reg. on Edu. for Persons w/ Disabilities	Pathways to the Future		2001 ECD White Paper
Convention on the Rights of Persons with Disabilities (2006)						
Views persons with disabilities as capable individuals who are knowledgeable of their rights, and are active members of society	Ratified	Drafted and Supported	Ratified	Ratified	Ratified	Ratified

**Provincial governments, not federal, regulate education in Canada
*1990 BPDP Law = 1990 Law of the People's Republic of China on the Basic Protection of Disabled Persons
*** 1995 Law on Social Protection of People with Disabilities

Figure 3.1 The key aspects of policies related to early childhood intervention and the approaches to these policies taken by Brazil, Canada, China, New Zealand, Russia, and South Africa.

service coordination among the relevant government departments and nonprofit services, with public or nongovernmental agencies intervening only when necessary (Stout, 2009).

COUNTRY MATRIX

Figure 3.1 outlines the key aspects of policies related to early childhood intervention and the approaches to these policies taken by each of the countries examined in this chapter.

CONCLUSION

Children of all countries and ability levels are our future. They will make decisions that keep nations at peace or bring us to war. They will discover cures for disease, invent new technology for good or evil, and raise future generations. Therefore, all countries will benefit from awareness of global policies and programs that improve children's opportunities and help them progress personally, academically, and socially so that they succeed in life. Furthermore, this information would be an asset in countries where policy and practice for children with special needs has not developed or been implemented to the standards proposed by international human rights agreements. This is clearly recommended in the Convention on the Rights of Children, where Part Four of Article 23 states that all countries supporting the CRC should engage in the open sharing of knowledge and best practices for the care of children with disabilities, with the intention of enhancing the capacity of underresourced countries (UNOHCHR, 1990; UNICEF, 2008).

This chapter reviews international laws and policies to provide a foundation for fair and equal treatment of all children. Yet, as evident in the country profile section, there is vast diversity in supports and services available to children, especially children with special needs. This discrepancy among nations challenges professionals to work across cultures to develop standards of care and service for these children. We can begin by creating a common language of terms, definitions, measurements, and standards to identify children in need and raise their education, health care, and welfare to the forefront of the political agendas of their countries.

REFERENCES

Asia-Pacific Development Center on Disability. (2002). *Country Profile: People's Republic of China*. Retrieved from Statistical Data on Disability Profile, http://www.apcdfoundation.org/?q=content/china

Asmal, K. (2001a). Education white paper 5 on early childhood education. Meeting the challenge of early childhood development in South Africa. Ministry of Education.

Asmal, K. (2001b). Address at the Launch of the White Paper for Early Childhood Development and the Nation-wide Audit of ECD Provisioning in South Africa. Ministry of Education

Ballard, K. (1996). Inclusive education in New Zealand: Culture, context and ideology. *Cambridge Journal of Education, 26*(1).

Bascand, G. (2006). 2006 Disability Survey.

Burns, K. K., & Gordon, G. L. (2009). Analyzing the impact of disability legislation in Canada and the United States. *Journal of Disability Policy Studies* published online Nov. 30, 2009.

Celia, S. (2004). Interventions with infants and families at risk: Context and culture. *Infant Mental Health, 25*(5): 502–507.

Chen, Y. (1996). *China Policy on Inclusive Education*. Beijing, China: National Institute for Educational Research.

China Disabled Persons' Federation. (2006). *Communique on major statistics of the Second China National Sample Survey on Disability*. Retrieved from http://www.cdpf.org.cn/old/english/top-7.htm

Dalziel, H. L. (2001). *The New Zealand disability strategy making a world of difference*. Whakanui Oranga, New Zealand Ministry of Health.

Deng, M. & Poon-McBrayer, K. F. (2004). Inclusive Education in China: Conceptualisation and Realization. *Asia-Pacific Journal of Education, 24*(2), 143–157.

Disability Rights Education and Defense Fund, Seventh National People's Congress. (1986). *Compulsory education law of the People's Republic of China*. Congress, People's Republic of China: Law Publishers.

Disability Rights Education and Defense Fund, Seventh National People's Congress. (1990). *Law of the People's Republic of China on the Protection of Disabled Persons*. Congress, People's Republic of China: Legal System Publishers.

Eloff, I. J. (2006). Some thoughts on the perceptions of the role of educational psychologists in early childhood intervention. *Early Child Development and Care, 176* (2), 111–127.

Epstein, I. (1992). Special education issues in China's modernization. In R. Hayhoe (Ed.), *Education and modernization: The Chinese experience*. Elmsford, NY: Pergamon.

Freitas, L. B. B., Shelton, T. L., & Tudge, J. R. H. (2008). Conceptions of US and Brazilian early childhood care and education: A historical and comparative analysis. *International Journal of Behavioral Development, 32*, 161.

Friendly, M. J. (2007). *Early Childhood Education and Care in Canada 2006* (7th ed.).

Gargiulo, R., &. Piao, Y. (1996). Early childhood special education in the People's Republic of China. *Early Child Development and Care, 118*, 35–43.

Government, of Canada. (2008). Human Resources and Skills Development. Advancing the Inclusion of People with Disabilities.

Government of Canada. (2009). *Canada's Universal Child Care Plan*. Retrieved April 1, 2009, from http://www.universalchildcare.ca/eng/why_ucc/index .shtml

Government of Canada Federal. (2004). *Federal/Provincial/Territorial Communiqué on Early Childhood Development*. Retrieved from http://www.ecd-elcc.ca/en/ ecd/ecd_home.shtml

Governmental Report. (1994). *On childhood conditions in the Russian Federation*. (Gosudarstvennyy Doklad "O polozhenii detey v Rossiyskoy Federatsii"). Moscow.

Kamerman, S. B. (2000). Early Childhood Intervention Policies: An International Perspective. In J. P. Shonkoff & S. J. Meisels (Eds.), *Handbook of early childhood intervention*. Cambridge: Cambridge University Press.

Liddell, C. A., & Kemp, J. (1995). Providing services for young children in South Africa. *International Journal of Educational Development, 15*(1), 71–78.

Lumpkin, H. G., & Aranha, M. S. F. (2003). The right to a good and supportive start in life. In S. L. Odom, M. J. Hanson, & J. A. Blackman (Eds.), *Early intervention practices around the world*. Baltimore: Paul H. Brookes.

Malofeev, N. N. (1996). *Spetsialnoye obrazovaniye v Rossii i za rubezhom*. (*Special education in Russia and abroad*). Moscow: Institute for Special Education.

Malofeev, N. N. (2000). *Sovremennyy etap v razvitii sistemy spetsialnogo obrazovaniya v Rossii: rezultaty issledovaniya kak osnova dlya postroyeniya programmy razvitiya.* (*The current stage in the development of special education in Russia: results of the study as a basis for building programs*). Moscow: Almanac ICP RAO 1-2000.

Max Bell Foundation. (2006). *What is early intervention?* Retrieved March 26, 2009, from http://www.earlyinterventioncanada.com/early_intervention.html

McCabe, H. (2003). The beginnings of inclusion in the People's Republic of China. *Research and Practice for Persons with Severe Disabilities, 28*(1), 16–22.

McClain, C., Howell, C., Lagadien, F., Pretorius, L., Rantho, M., & Thompson, P. (1997). Integrated National Disability Strategy White Paper. Office of the President.

McGill University & Yaldei Development Center. (2006). Canadian data. From http://www.earlyinterventioncanada.com/pdf/PopulationData.pdf

McLoughlin, C., Zhou, Z., & Clark, E. (2005). Reflections on the development and status of contemporary special education services in China. *Psychology in the Schools, 42*(3), 273–283.

Mont, D. (2007). *Measuring disability prevalence*. World Bank Disability and Development Team.

Muhamedrahimov, R. J. (2000). New attitudes: Infant care facilities in Saint-Petersburg (Russia). In J. D. Osofsky & H. E. Fitzgerald (Eds.), *WAIMH handbook of infant mental health. Vol.1: Perspectives on infant mental health* (pp. 245–294). New York: John Wiley & Sons.

New Zealand Ministry of Health. (2000). *The New Zealand Public Health and Disability Act 2000*.

New Zealand Office of Disability Issues. (2008a). *The New Zealand Disability Strategy: Common questions*. Retrieved from http://www.odi.govt.nz/nzds/ common-questions.html

New Zealand Office of Disability Issues. (2008b). *The New Zealand Disability Strategy: Progress reports*. Retrieved from http://www.odi.govt.nz/nzds/progress -reports/index.html

New Zealand Office of Disability Issues. (2009). *The New Zealand Disability Strategy: History of the Strategy*. Retrieved from http://www.odi.govt.nz/nzds/strategy-history.html

New Zealand Statistics. (2006). Table Builder. 2006 Disability Survey, Statistics New Zealand.

Odom, S. (2003). *Early intervention practices around the world*. Baltimore: Paul H. Brookes.

Pang, Y. A. (2006). The development of special education in China. *International Journal of Special Education, 2*(1), 77–86.

Peters, R. D. (2000). *Developing capacity and competence in the better beginnings, better futures communities: Short-term findings report*. Kingston, Ontario.

Peters, R. D. (2004). *Better beginnings, better futures: A comprehensive, community-based project for early childhood development. Highlights of Lessons Learned*. Kingston, Ontario.

Policy Brief of the Russian Academy of Education to the Government of the Russian Federation. (2007). *Modernizatsiya sistemy spetsialnogo obrazovaniya v RF: Dostizheniya, problemy, perspektivy. ("Modernization of the special education system in Russia: Achievements, problems and perspectives")*. Following the meeting, Bureau of the Department of psychology of Russian Academy of Education. Moscow, February 21.

Razenkova, Y. A. (2009). Predlozheniya po effektivnomu ispolzovaniyu organizatsionnykh mekhanizmov dlya sovershenstvovaniya i razvitiya sistemy ranney pomoshchi v razlichnykh regionakh strany. (Proposals to effective use of organizational mechanisms for perfection and development of early support system in various regions of the country). *Defektologiya, 4,* 61–64.

Saloojee, G., Phohole, M., Saloojee, H., & Ijsselmuiden, C. (2006). Unmet health, welfare and educational needs of disabled children in an impoverished South African peri-urban township. *Child: Care, Health and Development, 33*(3), 230–235.

Stout, B. (2009). Residential care in South Africa. In M. E. Courtney & D. Iwaniec (Eds.), *Residential Care of Children*. Oxford: Oxford University Press.

Stratford, B., & Ng, H. (2000). People with disabilities in China: Changing outlook—new solutions—growing problems. *International Journal of Disability, Development and Education, 47*(1), 7–14.

Telyukov, A., & Paterson, M. (2009). Assessment of USAID's child welfare programs in Russia. Evaluation Report. Gaithersburg, MD: Terra P. Group.

Tsai-Hsing, H., McCabe, H., & Bao-Jen, L. (2003). Cultural issues and service provision in rural areas. In In S. L. Odom, M. J. Hanson, J. A. Blackman, & S. Kaul (Eds.), *Early intervention practices around the world*. Baltimore: Paul H. Brookes.

United Nations. (1948). *The Universal Declaration of Human Rights*. Retrieved March 25, 2009, from http://www.un.org/Overview/rights.html

United Nations Children's Fund (UNICEF). (2005). Revised country programme document: Russian Federation. Retrieved from http://www.unicef.org/about/execboard/files/Russia_CPD_English(1).pdf

United Nations Children's Fund (UNICEF). (2007). UNICEF: A human rights based approach to education for all. New York: United Nations Children's Fund/United Nations Educational, Scientific and Cultural Organization.

United Nations Children's Fund (UNICEF). (2008). *Convention on the Rights of the Child*. Retrieved from http://www.unicef.org/crc/index_30160.html

United Nations Children's Fund (UNICEF). (2009). *I have the right: UNICEF Russia launches child rights campaign.* Retrieved from http://www.unicef.org/infoby country/russia_51631.html

United Nations Educational Scientific and Cultural Organization (UNESCO). (1960). Convention against discrimination in education. Retrieved from http://www.unesco.org/education/pdf/DISCRI_E.PDF

United Nations Educational Scientific and Cultural Organization (UNESCO). (2006). International Bureau of Education. South Africa Early Childhood Care and Education (ECCE) Programmes. Retrieved October 30, 2009, from http://unesdoc.unesco.org/images/0014/001472/147241e.pdf

United Nations Educational Scientific and Cultural Organization (UNESCO). (2007.) Education for All by 2015: Will we make it? Retrieved from http://unesdoc.unesco.org/images/0015/001547/154743e.pdf.

United Nations Educational Scientific and Cultural Organization (UNESCO). (2009). *Education.* Retrieved from http://portal.unesco.org/education/en/ev.php-URL_ID=48712&URL_DO=DO_TOPIC&URL_SECTION=201.html

United Nations Enable Convention on the Rights of Persons with Disabilities. Retrieved from http://www.un.org/disabilities/default.asp?navid=12&pid=150

United Nations Enable Convention on the Rights of Persons with Disabilities. *The International Year of Disabled Persons 1981.* Retrieved from http://www.un.org/esa/socdev/enable/disiydp.htm

United Nations Enable Convention on the Rights of Persons with Disabilities. (1976). *Promoting the rights of persons with disabilities.* Retrieved from http://www.un.org/esa/socdev/enable/rights/humanrights.htm

United Nations Enable Convention on the Rights of Persons with Disabilities. (1982). *World Programme of Action Concerning Disabled Persons.* Retrieved from http://www.un.org/disabilities/default.asp?id=23

United Nations Enable Convention on the Rights of Persons with Disabilities. (1993). *The Standard Rules on the Equalization of Opportunities for Persons with Disabilities.* Retrieved from http://www.un.org/esa/socdev/enable/dissre00.htm

United Nations Office of the High Commissioner for Human Rights. (1975). *The Declaration on the Rights of Disabled Persons.* Retrieved from http://www.unhchr.ch/html/menu3/b/72.htm

United Nations Office of the High Commissioner for Human Rights [UNOHCHR]. (1990). *Convention on the Rights of the Child.* Retrieved from http://www2.ohchr.org/english/law/crc.htm

United States Central Intelligence Agency. (2009a). *World Factbook: Brazil.* Retrieved from https://www.cia.gov/library/publications/the-world-factbook/geos/br.html

United States Central Intelligence Agency. (2009b). *World Factbook: Canada.* Retrieved June 4, 2009, from https://www.cia.gov/library/publications/the-world-factbook/geos/ca.html

United States Central Intelligence Agency. (2009c). *World Factbook: China.* Retrieved from https://www.cia.gov/library/publications/the-world-factbook/geos/ch.html

United States Central Intelligence Agency. (2009d). *World Factbook: Russia.* Retrieved from https://www.cia.gov/library/publications/the-world-factbook/geos/rs.html

United States Central Intelligence Agency. (2009e). *World Factbook: South Africa.* Retrieved from https://www.cia.gov/library/publications/the-world-factbook/geos/sf.html

United States Department of State. (2008). *Background Note: Canada.* Retrieved from http://www.state.gov/r/pa/ei/bgn/2089.htm

Walton, E., Nel, N., Hugo, A., & Muller, H. (2009). The extent and practice of inclusion in independent schools in South Africa. *South African Journal of Education, 29,* 105–126.

World Health Organization. (2005). *International Classification of Functioning, Disability and Health (ICF).* Retrieved from http://www.who.int/classifications/icf/en

World Health Organization Regional Office for Europe. (2005). *Declaration on the Rights of Disabled Persons.* Retrieved from http://www.euro.who.int/mental health/declarations/20061204_1

Zhao, L., Guo, C. F., & Zhou, M. (1997). The implementation of counterpart activities for healthy young children and young children who are deaf. In Y. Chen, *Theory and practice of the reform of China's integrated education* (pp. 198–202). Beijing: Xinhua Chubanshe.

Chapter 4

Reflections on Early Identification

Bruce K. Shapiro

A developmental disability is a severe, chronic disability attributable to mental and/or physical impairments that are likely to continue indefinitely, resulting in substantial functional limitations in three or more life activity areas: self-care, receptive and expressive language, learning, mobility, self-direction, capacity for independent living, and economic self-sufficiency. These disorders disclose themselves before age 22 and require care, treatment, or other services of lifelong or extended duration. Children younger than age 9 may be considered to have a developmental disability without showing limitations in three or more life activity areas if they have a high likelihood of meeting those criteria in later life without services and supports (Public Law 106-402, 2000).

Please be aware that different states in the United States may use different definitions in state law for the term developmental disability. Table 4.1 lists the definitions of the developmental disabilities.

Developmental disabilities are a group of conditions that are due to abnormal brain function or to metabolism or degenerative processes. They limit typical activities. The disorders outlined in Table 4.1 are defined by the nature of the limitation. The degree of the limitation, the process that results in the limitation, or the cause of the brain malfunction is not required for the diagnosis. However, understanding the underlying brain malfunction is important. Brain malfunction in childhood can result from many causes. Genetic disorders, infection, nutritional and metabolic disorders, trauma, hypoxia (lack of oxygen) or ischemia (lack of blood flow), and toxins (tobacco, lead, alcohol) are some of the more common etiologies of brain malfunction. These causes may give rise to widespread brain malfunction that result in multiple diagnoses for children with developmental disabilities. For example, many children with cerebral palsy also have epilepsy and intellectual disability. It is the multiple combinations of disorders of

Table 4.1   Developmental Disabilities: Definitions and Prevalence

Attention Deficit Hyperactivity Disorder (ADHD): ADHD is a brain disorder that is characterized by developmentally inappropriate levels of inattention, distractibility, impulsivity, and hyperactivity. Many children with ADHD will not meet the full criteria for developmental disabilities, but those who are more severely affected will. The prevalence of ADHD is between 5% and 8% of school-aged children.

Autism: Autism is a brain development disorder that is characterized by impaired social interaction and communication and by restricted and repetitive behavior. Children who do not manifest these characteristics by age 3 or who do not fully meet the diagnostic criteria for autism are called "autism spectrum disorder." Approximately 1% of children have autism spectrum disorder.

Blindness: Best corrected visual acuity of 20/400 or less or restricted field of vision to 10 degrees. The prevalence of legal blindness is 0.07%.

Cerebral Palsy (CP): CP is a disorder of movement or posture that is due to a brain disorder or defect that occurs in the developing fetal or infant brain. The disorder does not worsen, but the symptoms may change as the child ages. The prevalence of cerebral palsy is 0.1–0.3% of children.

Deafness: There is no uniformly accepted threshold for deafness. The term "deaf" is sometimes used to describe someone who has an approximately 90 dB or greater hearing loss or who cannot use hearing to process speech and language information, even with the use of hearing aids. The prevalence of communicatively handicapping hearing loss (moderate to profound) is 0.1–0.2% in the general population.

Epilepsy: Epilepsy is a brain disorder involving repeated, spontaneous seizures of any type. The prevalence of epilepsy in children is 0.4–0.9%.

Intellectual Disability: Significantly sub-average general intellectual function accompanied by deficits in adaptive behavior that commences before 18 years of age. The prevalence of intellectual disability is approximately 1.2%.

Receptive Expressive Language Disorder: This is a group of disorders distinguished by the child's inability to understand language or express it. A child with mixed receptive expressive language disorder is not able to communicate thoughts, needs, or wants at the same level or with the same complexity as his or her peers. They have difficulty understanding what is being said to them and often have a smaller vocabulary than their peers. Receptive Expressive Language Disorder is found in about 3% of school-aged children.

Specific Learning Disabilities (Including Dyslexia): "A disorder in one or more of the basic psychological processes involved in understanding or in using language, spoken or written, which may manifest in the imperfect ability to listen, think, speak, read, write, spell, or do mathematical calculations" (PL 108-446, 2004). Many children with specific learning disabilities will not meet the full criteria for developmental disabilities, but those who are more severely affected will. The prevalence of specific learning disabilities is 5% of the school-aged population.

Source: Prevalence statistics derived from Centers for Disease Control and Prevention, National Center on Birth Defects and Developmental Disabilities Web site.

varying degrees that call for individualized treatment programs for people with developmental disabilities.

Understanding that brain malfunction shows itself in many ways may be useful for early identification. A child with a developmental dysfunction in one area is likely to have a developmental dysfunction in another area. As an example, children who are late walkers often have disordered language development.

EARLY IDENTIFICATION

What Is Early Identification?

Early identification is the prelude to early intervention. The object of early identification is to identify a disorder at a stage before it is fully evident and to undertake interventions that will either prevent or substantially modify the natural progression of the disorder. Identification is not an end, but the beginning of a process that leads to the provision of care and, hopefully, a better outcome for the child.

Early identification seeks to detect children who are likely to have a disorder and enables further evaluation to determine whether the disorder is present. Early identification describes a series of techniques that result in diagnosis. Methods used for early identification range from using public service advertisements on radio and television to reach the general population, to the measurement of biochemical processes in the body fluids of an individual. Defining conditions that place one at greater risk for developmental disability and assessing/evaluating those at risk are other means that might be employed.

Why Is Early Identification Beneficial?

The justification for early identification is that it leads to better outcomes for the child. Basically, early identification is the first step in the therapeutic process. Early identification facilitates evaluation, assessment, and diagnosis and leads to early intervention.

Early identification may allow for interventions that cure or prevent a disorder. Some disorders that previously damaged the developing brain can now be treated and developmental disability averted. This is the justification for newborn bloodspot screening (see below). In the case of metabolic disorders, such as congenital hypothyroidism or phenylketonuria, supplying deficient hormones or applying a special diet prevents the developmental dysfunction associated with these disorders in the past.

Early intervention may alter the character and severity of the developmental disorder. There is a general perception that starting therapy at an earlier age is associated with better outcomes. This is supported by studies that show that younger animals have increased ability to recover from brain injury (plasticity) and suggest critical periods (National Research Council and Institute of Medicine, 2000). However, the data that directly link the age that intervention commences and outcomes are few, and the studies have not consistently supported the assertion that earlier intervention results in better outcomes (Bruer, 1999).

Early identification leads to evaluation, assessment, and diagnosis. Establishing a diagnosis allows for development of a management program, enables long-term planning, and may lead to improved family functioning. Families often recognize developmental issues before the problem is identified by professionals. Many families experience substantial anxiety until a diagnosis is established and a management plan developed.

Secondary problems may result from failure to identify a developmental disorder. Children with cerebral palsy who maintain a fixed position may be at increased risk of scoliosis (i.e., curvature of the spine) and hip problems. Children with autism spectrum disorder may not respond to discipline in an expected fashion and may become severely anxious or aggressive. A child with vocal tic disorder may be misperceived as intentionally making noises to disrupt the class and gain attention. Early identification leads to recognition of the disorder, better understanding of its character, and utilization of treatments that minimize secondary problems.

Early identification holds the promise of developing interventions that are more effective than the ones that are used currently. Most of the interventions that are utilized for developmental disabilities were developed for older children and now are used for younger and younger children. The child who is identified at a younger age may be better served by a different treatment than those that have been established for older children. One example is the use of occupational therapy for young children with sensory integrative disorder and the use of cognitive behavioral therapy (CBT) for older children with the same symptom complex. Occupational therapy seeks to decrease the response to sensory stimuli by addressing the sensory systems directly; whereas cognitive behavioral therapy, as the name implies, uses cognitive and behavioral approaches to alter the response to sensory stimuli and requires children to be of an age such that they can understand and employ the techniques.

How Early Is Early?

This question is usually asked in an open-ended fashion. The implication is that if identification at 6 months is good, then identification at 5 months is better. The extension of that argument is that there is no limit to how early developmental disabilities can be identified. As a result, there could be no limit to the resources that would be expended on the identification process. Early identification becomes the end product and not a step in a process to early intervention.

Reframing the question to "How early is early enough?" results in an achievable outcome. "Enough" is a point at which substantial damage has not occurred and allows sufficient time for the rest of the processes to be implemented. It permits some flexibility in the system and allows for assessment and implementation of the intervention. Universal newborn screening programs (see below) have identification of hearing loss by one month as their goal but allow five more months for the confirmatory evaluation and intervention processes to be implemented.

Preconceptual Identification

Current technology allows for identification before conception for some disorders. Having this knowledge allows carriers of the conditions to make informed decisions about marriage and reproduction. It also allows for prenatal diagnosis. Two such examples are Fragile X syndrome and Tay-Sachs disease.

Fragile X syndrome is a chromosomal disorder that is the most commonly inherited form of intellectual disability in males and is found in approximately 8 percent of children with autism. Sisters of children with Fragile X syndrome may be screened to determine if they are carriers of the syndrome.

Tay-Sachs disease is an inherited disorder that causes a child's brain to lose function because of an enzyme deficiency. Approximately 1 in 30 Ashkenazi Jews have the gene for this disorder. Carriers of the disorder may be identified by a blood test.

Identification during Pregnancy

Many developmental disorders are the result of events that occur before delivery. Our abilities to detect developmental disorders in utero are limited, but this is an area of future growth. In-utero procedures may focus on delineating variations from normal pregnancy or focus on specific entities.

One example of procedures that are nonspecific is the non-stress test. The non-stress test is usually performed near the end of pregnancy. It may be used if there is concern about fetal well-being, if the mother has diabetes, if the fetus has not grown as well as expected, or if the pregnancy is extending beyond term. The non-stress test measures the fetal heart rate when the fetus is moving and compares it to the heart rate when the fetus is resting. A reactive non-stress test means that the blood flow to the fetus is adequate. A nonreactive non-stress test suggests that the fetus may be at risk.

A number of blood tests may be used in the first or second trimester to detect spina bifida/anencephaly or Down syndrome and other chromosomal disorders. Amniocentesis and chorionic villus sampling are techniques that obtain amniotic fluid or a piece of the placenta so that genetic and metabolic studies can be performed. Ultrasound is used to determine the number of fetuses, assess fetal growth, and identify structural abnormalities such as hydrocephalus or urological abnormalities. Fetal MRI imaging is a relatively new procedure that is increasingly used in clinical settings to augment the information provided by ultrasound.

Neonatal Identification

Newborn screening has expanded as new technologies have been developed. For example, at present, the state of Maryland screens newborns for hearing loss and 54 rare diseases. Blood samples are collected on filter paper and sent to the state laboratory for analysis. The diseases screened include disorders of the metabolism of amino acids, organic acids, urea cycle, fatty acid oxidation, carbohydrates, hormones, hemoglobin, and cystic fibrosis. (See State of Maryland Family Health Administration [http://fha.maryland.gov/pdf/genetics/Pamphlet_NBS.pdf] for details.) Most of these disorders can be effectively managed if detected early. For information on your state law, see http://www.ncsl.org/IssuesResearch/Health/NewbornGeneticand MetabolicScreeningLaws/tabid/14416/Default.aspx

Postnatal Identification

The most common techniques used to identify developmental disabilities are (1) risk registries, (2) population screening, and

Table 4.2   Calculation of Sensitivity and Specificity

	Disorder Present	Disorder Absent
Test Positive	A	C
Test Negative	B	D
Total	A + B	C + D
Sensitivity is A/(A + B)		
Specificity is D/(C + D)		

(3) developmental failure/maternal referral. Each of these techniques attempts to classify children as being more or less likely to have a developmental disability. The ideal approach to early identification would identify all of the children with developmental disabilities in the most efficient manner. The likelihood ratios that describe the efficiency of classification are sensitivity and specificity. Sensitivity is the ability to correctly identify children with the disorder of interest. Specificity is the ability to correctly identify children who do not have the disorder of interest (see Table 4.2).

The American Academy of Pediatrics (AAP) endorses instruments that have sensitivity and specificity abilities of 70–80 percent. Using a hypothetical instrument with those classification abilities and applying to a population of 10,000 children who have a 1 percent rate of a disorder would yield Table 4.3. The results show that for each positive test, only 31 percent of children will have the disorder. This means that almost twice as many confirmatory evaluations are required. For each negative test, 97 percent of children will not have the disorder, but 3 percent of children would. Depending on the disorder, this could be a very meaningful shortcoming of the method used. Overall, 20 percent of children will be misclassified.

Table 4.3   Illustration of the Performance of a Hypothetical Instrument

	Disorder Present	Disorder Absent
Test Positive	800	1,800
Test Negative	200	7,200
Total	1,000	9,000

Risk

Risk is a statistical concept that says that a person is more or less likely to have a condition. Risk may be based on group status or by performance. An example of the former is being born prematurely with a birth weight less than 1,500 grams, while an example of the latter is not walking until 20 months.

When risk is assigned, it is most often relative risk. Relative risk compares the frequency of a disorder seen in people who have been exposed to a condition to the frequency of the disorder in people who have not been exposed to the condition. For example, the National Perinatal Collaborative Project (NPCP) was a longitudinal research project that followed approximately 50,000 women's pregnancies from identification until the children were 7½ years old. Perinatal refers to the time from the fifth month of pregnancy until one month after birth. Extensive data were collected on the mother's pregnancies, perinatal period, and the child's early development. One factor, the overall impression of brain abnormality at the time of discharge from the hospital, carried a 99-fold increased risk of cerebral palsy at age 7.

While the first impression is that this is a strongly predictive factor, further analysis suggests otherwise (Shapiro & Gwynn, 2008). First, this factor occurred rarely in the study population. Only 1.2 percent of the population had the factor. Second, most of the children with cerebral palsy did not have the factor. Only 23 percent of the children with cerebral palsy had the factor. Third, the factor predicted other outcomes more than the targeted outcome. Fifty-three percent of those who had the factor died before age 7. Finally, high relative risk for conditions that occur infrequently does not predict the presence of the disorder well. Of the children in the NPCP, the prevalence of cerebral palsy at age 7 was 0.153 percent (1.53 in 1,000). Applying the relative risk of 99-fold meant that 15 percent of the children who had the factor manifested cerebral palsy at age 7 (99 × 0.153%). It also means that 85 percent did not. Establishing a treatment program based on relative risk is destined to be successful because most children do not demonstrate the condition they are "at risk" of developing. This is why we sometimes think treatment strategies have worked because they were "treating" something that did not exist.

Risk Registries

Risk registries identify children as "at risk" when they have characteristics that are associated with the disorder of interest. Most risk registries use historic risk to identify children who require evaluations to confirm the diagnosis. They are used because the risk factors are easily identified—for example, birth weight less than 1,500 grams—but they are limited when applied to individuals. First, as noted above, most children do not have the condition that they are "at risk" of having. In addition, most children with developmental disabilities do not come from an "at risk" population. While prematurity is associated with cerebral palsy, most cerebral palsy is found in children who were delivered at full term. Similarly, while Down syndrome is associated with advanced maternal age, most children with Down syndrome are born to mothers less than 35 years old.

Expanding risk registries beyond the most basic information may prove challenging. Some risk factors may be difficult to define, such as hyperactivity or colic. Some factors may have poor classification abilities (sensitivity and specificity) and poorly distinguish those with the condition of interest (e.g., teenage pregnancy). Some risk factors may not exert their effect directly, or may do so on many different levels. For example, low socioeconomic status is associated with developmental disability, but the mechanisms by which low socioeconomic status causes developmental disability remain to be defined. Finally, risk registries can be expanded to the point that they cannot be implemented. To establish a risk registry that focuses on prematurity would require evaluating approximately 10 percent of the population.

Risk registries established on the basis of performance are more likely to better classify children who are at risk for developmental disabilities because performance-based classification is more specific than risk assigned by historical risk. Performance-based registries require more initial effort than historic risk registries because a larger number of children need to have their performance evaluated. However, the total effort expended might be less because fewer children would require confirmatory evaluations based on performance rather than group status. Assigning risk based on performance is the foundation for screening.

Screening

Screening is the application of procedures to a population without symptoms to identify people who have a high likelihood of having the disorder of interest. Screening is the first step in the diagnostic process. Screening does not yield a diagnosis. The result of screening is "risk." A child who "fails" a screen requires an evaluation to confirm the disorder. Even the biochemical tests performed as part of the newborn screening require confirmatory testing before treatment is initiated.

Screening is justified if the condition will benefit from early diagnosis and treatment and that the cost-benefit ratio is positive. This assumes that the condition exists without symptoms or that early intervention will alter the natural history of the disorder. To accomplish this assumes that the condition of interest can be identified in measurable terms and that the instruments used to screen have acceptable psychometric properties. Finally, for screening to be justified, diagnostic and treatment services must be available to confirm the screen results.

The American Academy of Pediatrics has developed a system of surveillance and screening to guide the identification processes (AAP Council on Children with Disabilities et al., 2006). Surveillance is a flexible, longitudinal, continuous, and cumulative process whereby knowledgeable health care professionals identify children who may have developmental problems. Screening is used at 9, 18, and 30 months, or if surveillance raises questions. The tests that are recommended are listed in Table 4.4 and are widely available. Other groups may recommend different instruments. Other instruments exist but were not recommended because of their screening characteristics. This system is being implemented, and data about the efficacy of this process should be forthcoming in the near future.

Developmental Failure

Developmental disabilities present in many different ways, but the way they come to attention is not random. Many of these presentations are readily observed by early childhood personnel. They include the most common ones of abnormal physical appearance, physiological instability, poor interaction with the environment, motor or language delays, behavioral disturbances, and poor school performance. What these wide ranges of presenting symptoms have in common is that they represent failure to meet age-appropriate expectations. The age at which it is recognized that appropriate expectations are not being met is closely related to the child's ultimate diagnosis (Lock, Shapiro, Ross, & Capute, 1986). Table 4.5 lists the age-related developmental expectations. Parents identify most children with developmental disabilities. They raise concerns when children do not meet age-appropriate expectations. Mothers observe their children and compare them to the children of friends, neighbors, relatives, and play groups. By the time a mother has decided that her child is not meeting age-appropriate expectations, she has conducted a study that controls for

Table 4.4   Developmental Screening Tools Endorsed by the AAP

General Developmental Screening Tools

  Ages and Stages Questionnaires
  Battelle Developmental Inventory Screening Tool, 2nd ed.
  Bayley Infant Neurodevelopmental Screener
  Brigance Screens-II
  Child Development Inventory
  Child Development Review-Parent Questionnaire
  Denver-II Developmental Screening Test
  Infant Development Inventory
  Parents' Evaluation of Developmental Status

Language and Cognitive Screening Tools

  The Capute Scales
  Communication and Symbolic Behavior Scales-Developmental Profile
  Early Language Milestone Scale

Motor Screening Tools

  Early Motor Pattern Profile
  Motor Quotient

Autism Screening Tools

  The Checklist for Autism in Toddlers
  Modified Checklist for Autism in Toddlers
  Pervasive Developmental Disorders Screening Test-II
  1. Primary Care Screener
  2. Developmental Clinic Screener
  Screening Tool for Autism in Two-Year-Olds
  Social Communication Questionnaire

Source: AAP Council on Children with Disabilities et al., 2006.

all the demographic and Table 4.5 confounding variables. Mothers cannot only identify children who are substantially different, but they can also estimate their child's functional level with great accuracy (Pulsifer, Hoon, Palmer, Gopalan, & Capute, 1994).

Assessment

Risk registries, screening, and recognition of developmental delay are techniques that place a child "at risk." They are the first steps in the diagnostic process. Assessment takes the process beyond assignment of "risk" to diagnosis.

Diagnosis is of major importance with developmental disabilities. Diagnosis facilitates treatment. It defines the parameters of the treatment and allows goals to be established. Diagnosis allows prognosis.

Table 4.5   Age-Related Developmental Expectations

Age	Function	Questions
Newborn	Cute	Whom does he look like?
	Major organ systems work	
2–6 Months	Interacts with the environment	Does she see?
		Does she hear?
		Does she recognize you?
6–15 Months	Motor achievement	Does he sit, crawl, walk?
18–30 Months	Language achievement	How many words does she have?
		Is she intelligible?
30–48 Months	Fine motor	Is she overactive?
	Behavior	How well does she play?
	Self-help skills	What is the quality of her work—cutting, coloring, pasting?
		Can she feed, dress, or toilet by herself?

Source: Modified from Shapiro & Gwynn (2008).

Understanding the nature and potential outcomes of a disorder enables the long-term planning that is critical to successful management programs. A specific diagnosis is required to determine the cause of the developmental disability. If an etiology can be determined, then research may enhance understanding of the disorder and open the possibilities of effective treatments or prevention of the disorder for future children. Diagnosis is important for planning and the development of policy. Knowing the number of children with condition X enables planners to determine the services that are required in the community to meet the needs of those families.

Developmental Assessment

The purpose of developmental assessment is to establish a diagnosis, delineate other disorders, and generate hypotheses about the possible causes of the dysfunction. While there are many tools for assessing development, the basic principles derive from the work of Arnold Gesell.

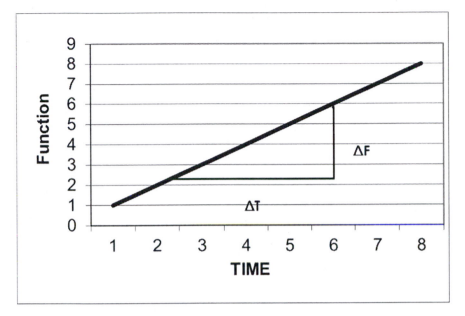

Figure 4.1   Developmental quotients compare the age of achievement (functional age) to chronological age.

   Gesell developed an empirical system of developmental assessment that was based on his observations of children (Gesell & Amatruda, 1947). Gesell held that development was an extension of neurological function, and that if a child was developing normally, the brain was functioning normally, or that the compensatory mechanisms were working. He noted that development did not occur randomly. Children followed an ordered sequence—in the motor area they rolled, sat, crawled, and then walked. One of his most important observations was that children who were delayed followed the same sequences, but their achievements occurred at a later age. Gesell's definition of developmental sequences or milestones could be described as rates that compared the age of achievement to chronological age. This was called developmental quotient. For example, a 3-year-old who has achieved an 18-month level would have a developmental quotient of 50 percent (18 months/36 months = 50%).

   Delay is what brings children to the attention of caregivers. (For a listing of developmental disabilities, including definitions and prevalence, see Figure 4.1.) The definition of delay may be arbitrary and may be established by the state (P.L.108-446, 2004). Traditionally it

Table 4.6   Developmental Dissociation

	Gross motor	Fine Motor/ Problem Solving	Language	Personal- Social
Cerebral Palsy	Decreased	±	±	±
Intellectual Disability	±	Decreased	Decreased	Decreased
Receptive Expressive Language Disorder or Hearing Loss	±	±	Decreased	±
Autism Spectrum	±	±	Decreased	Decreased

Table of dissociation: ± does not always imply typical development. It refers to relative sparing of this domain of development. Delay may be in ± areas but not to the degree that is "decreased."

was a quotient of 70 percent or less (two standard deviations if 100 was the average and a standard deviation was 15 points). Some practitioners felt that one standard deviation (DQ of 85 or less) would merit attention. Current practice uses 75 percent. Development may be asynchronous, meaning that different aspects of development such as gross motor, fine motor (hand function), problem solving, language, and personal-social (activities of daily living, play) may develop at different rates. These differences in development can be used to achieve early diagnosis. Developmental quotients can be calculated for each aspect of development. Differences of more than 15 percent are significant. Table 4.6 demonstrates developmental dissociation. Of particular note is the primacy of delayed language in developmental disabilities.

Finally, deviation from the sequence is not typical. This may be seen in children who violate the developmental sequence, as in the case of walking before crawling. Deviance may also be noted in children who evidence uncoupled development. They do some things that are age appropriate but not others (e.g., the child who has 75 words but does not use spontaneous two-word phrases). Deviance is often noted in autism spectrum disorder.

Uses of Developmental Milestones

Developmental assessment is a system used to define development in children. The ability of developmental assessment to diagnose and

Table 4.7   Developmental Milestones

Language Milestones	
First word	11 months
Second word	12 months
Third word	13 months
4–6 words	15 months
7–10 words	17 months
50 words	21 months
Two-word phrases	21 months
Gross Motor Milestones	
Roll tummy to back	4 months
Roll back to tummy	5 months
Sits alone	6 months
Crawls	8 months
Walks	12 months

Source: Adapted from Shapiro & Gwynn (2008).

predict outcomes is based on the milestones chosen, the precision with which they are applied, and the child's degree of delay. Deviations from what is typical are predicted with much greater accuracy than degrees of normality. Developmental assessment cannot predict whether, or which, college a child will attend.

Developmental milestones are not equal in their ability to predict. To be useful, milestones must be observed with ease. They must be present in most of the population. They have to appear within a narrow time frame (milestones that occur between 4 and 14 months [a 10-month span] are not useful for early identification). The milestones must be able to predict the disorder of interest.

Language milestones are most useful for the early diagnosis of intellectual disability, receptive-expressive language disorders, or autism spectrum disorders. Gross motor milestones include activities such as rolling, sitting, crawling, and cruising. They are important for the diagnosis of cerebral palsy. Given that many young children choose not to perform in the evaluation session, language, gross-motor, and personal-social milestones may be obtained historically by interviewing parents or other caregivers. Table 4.7 lists a number of language and motor milestones and their usual age of appearance.

Techniques of Milestone Usage

Developmental milestones may be used in many different ways. Milestones may be plotted on a graph. Ongoing monitoring and collection of milestone attainment allows for a curve to be developed that reflects the child's development. The curve shows changes in function (milestone achievement) over time (the child's age).

Criterion-referenced use of milestones is a cross-sectional sampling that samples behavior at a single point in time. Criteria-referenced methods hold the child's age or the function of interest constant. For example, a criterion-referenced use of milestones might ask that all children who were not walking (function) by 21 months (age) be further evaluated. Children who do not meet the criterion are identified for further evaluation. This is the mechanism of screening and does not result in a diagnosis.

Best performance is another method of cross-sectional sampling of a child's behavior. This technique is used by most standard evaluation instruments. A child is asked to perform on a test. The results, which reflect the child's performance at a single point in time, are compared to the performance of similarly aged children. Standard evaluation instruments assume that the child's performance on an assessment instrument is reflective of his abilities. Best performance allows both the age and function to vary.

Finally, retrospective analysis attempts to capture the dynamic aspects of development by sampling the age of achievement of several milestones and develop a summary quotient that reflects the child's development. For example, a child may have their first word at 22 months, have three words at 3 years, and start to use two-word phrases at 4 years. The developmental quotients are 50 percent (11/22), 42 percent (15/36), and 50 percent (24/48), respectively, leading one to conclude that the child is developing at about half of the typical rate. Using multiple milestones to derive a quotient improves diagnostic precision because it lessens the impact of single milestones.

Vision

Vision problems occur in 5 to 10 percent of preschoolers. While there are many different eye disorders, most fall into three categories: refractive error, strabismus, or amblyopia.

Refractive errors include nearsightedness (myopia), farsightedness (hyperopia), and astigmatism. Refractive errors rarely delay early development, save in extreme cases. Blindness is defined as best corrected visual acuity of less than 20/400 in the best eye or a field of vision that is restricted to 10 degrees. Blindness that is seen in infants and young children may be associated with other developmental disorders. Children who are blind often have residual visual ability, but blindness creates challenges for assessment in other developmental areas.

Strabismus, commonly called crossed or wandering eye, is a misalignment of the eyes. The misalignment may be intermittent or fixed. Strabismus occurs in approximately 2 to 4 percent of children. Early intervention for strabismus is important to prevent amblyopia.

Amblyopia is a loss of visual acuity due to brain suppression of the visual signal from an eye. It may be seen in strabismus that is not treated, where the visual signal from one eye is suppressed to prevent double vision. It may be seen as a result of marked differences in the visual acuity between the eyes. Rarely, amblyopia may result from obstruction of the visual signal coming into the eye, as in the case of a congenital cataract (deprivational amblyopia). Amblyopia may cause reduced vision to the level of functional blindness if the affected eye is untreated.

Visual screening commences in the newborn nursery. Newborn screening assesses the eye structures, responses to visual stimuli (such as eye closure to a bright light), and alignment. The ability to fix, follow objects, and alignment are the foci of the first few months. Ideally, this should be evaluated for each eye independently. The ability to see and obtain small objects (e.g., a piece of lint on the carpet) is appropriate for children in the first half-year of life.

Assessment of visual acuity that uses behavioral methods begins at 3 years of age, although estimates of visual acuity can be measured earlier. Techniques that measure pursuit of novel stimuli of graded sizes, or preferential looking, yield reliable measures of visual acuity but have not been widely adopted in the primary care setting.

The American Academy of Pediatrics Committee on Practice and Ambulatory Medicine (2003) endorsed the following tests for use in children who are 3 to 5 years of age: Snellen letters, Snellen numbers, Tumbling E, HOTV, and the Allen or LH test. The Tumbling E test requires the child to show which way the E is pointing. The HOTV tests uses letters that are more easily distinguished by preschool children because they are not affected by rotation. The Allen and LH tests are presented in picture format for children who do not know their letters. Asking younger children to match the stimuli they see to a testing board that contains all of the stimuli may increase their performance.

Details of specific visual screening tests have been reviewed recently (American Academy of Pediatrics Committee on Practice and Ambulatory Medicine, 2003; Tingley, 2007). Criteria for referral for additional evaluation include (1) structural abnormality at any age, (2) failure to show light appreciation in either eye at any age, (3) misalignment of the eyes, (4) visual acuity of 20/50 or worse or more than two lines difference between the eyes in 3-year olds, and (5) visual acuity of 20/40 or worse or more than two lines difference between the eyes in 4-year olds.

Screening for visual problems in preschool children is far from universal (Hartmann et al., 2006). A large multisite study revealed that successful screening for 3-year-olds was completed far less often than in 4-year olds (80% versus 94%). The authors also reported substantial variation in following the recommended protocol, referral rates, and follow-up. They concluded that all aspects of preschool vision screening need to be reviewed before an effective system can be achieved.

Hearing

Hearing loss may be viewed in several different ways. The nature of the hearing loss (conductive, sensorineural, mixed, or central), the degree of hearing loss, and the cause of the hearing loss are but several of the ways that hearing loss may be categorized.

Conductive hearing losses occur when sound is not transmitted to the hearing system. This type of hearing loss is quite common in preschool children and is associated with otitis media and fluid in the middle ear (effusion). The effusion blunts the transmittal of the sound signal and affects hearing. Conductive hearing losses are not usually permanent, but persistent effusions are treated by insertion of tympanostomy tubes. Although concern has been expressed about the relationship between persisting middle-ear effusions and developmental outcome, a number of studies have failed to show adverse developmental outcomes at school age in otherwise healthy children who have persisting middle-ear effusions (McCormick, Johnson, & Baldwin, 2006; Paradise et al., 2005).

Sensorineural hearing loss is the focus of universal newborn screening efforts. It is the type of hearing loss that affects the function of the auditory nerve. Sensorineural hearing loss may not be evident at birth and may develop later in childhood. Sensorineural hearing loss may have its onset after the newborn period, and it may progress as the child ages and becomes communicatively disabled. Consequently, sensorineural hearing losses require regular monitoring. Mixed hearing losses have elements of conductive and sensorineural dysfunction.

Central hearing loss is the result of the brain's inability to interpret the incoming sound stimuli. It does not affect the hearing apparatus. Landau Kleffner is a syndrome seen in preschool children that has language regression, seizures, central hearing loss, and atypical electroencephalogram as key components.

Hearing loss, like visual loss, may be categorized by the severity of the impairment. It is grouped by the loudness of the sound (dB) required to effect a response. Hearing loss may range from minimal (16–25 dB) to profound (more than 90 dB). Hearing loss in the moderate to profound range (more than 40 dB) occurs in 1 to 3/1,000 newborns.

There are many causes of hearing loss. Sensorineural hearing loss may result from infection, toxins, genetic, trauma, or structural causes (Nance, 2003; Roizen, 2003). Congenital cytomegalovirus infection (CMV), a viral infection that may be acquired during gestation, is a common cause of hearing loss. Some of the sensorineural hearing losses are associated with structural or functional abnormalities (e.g., Stickler syndrome or Alport syndrome), while others (e.g., connexin 26) are not.

The methods used for evaluating hearing are dependent on the ability of the child to cooperate. Physiologic measures, such as auditory brainstem responses or otoacoustic emissions, do not require the child's cooperation (see American Academy of Pediatrics, Joint Committee on Infant Hearing, 2007). Impedance audiometry provides useful information about the status of the middle ear and is used most often in the evaluation of conductive hearing loss. Visual reinforced audiometry may be used in children as young as 6 to 9 months to approximate hearing acuity. For those children who can be conditioned for visual reinforcement audiometry (VRA), the American Speech-Hearing-Language Association (ASHA) recommends screening with earphones to test each ear with 1,000, 2,000, and 4,000 Hz tones at 30 dB HL (American Speech-Language-Hearing Association, 1997). If the child cannot be conditioned to earphones, evaluation in sound field conditions may provide sufficient information to answer the question of whether the child has sufficient hearing for development of language. Conditioned play audiometry and use of headphones may be used in somewhat older children. For those children who can be conditioned for play audiometry (CPA), screening each ear (with 1,000, 2,000, and 4,000 Hz tones at 20 dB HL) is recommended. Referral should be made for children who show no response or no reliable response at level at 30 dB for VRA or 20 dB for CPA at any frequency in either ear.

Failed hearing screens are frequently seen in preschool children. In one study (Allen, Stuart, Everett, & Elangovan, 2004) only 54 percent of 3- and 4-year-old children who attended passed the initial screening that included pure tone audiometry, impedance tympanometry, and direct visualization of the ear drum and external structures (otoscopy). About 30 percent of children failed pure tone audiometry. Thirty percent of study children also failed impedance tympanometry. After a rescreening, 76 percent of children passed. Follow-up assessment compliance after the rescreening was poor, approximating 10 percent. The hearing status of 18.3 percent of the eligible children was never ascertained. While the number of failed screens was high, the number of children with confirmed hearing loss was not. Of the children who completed the audiologic screening and/or received diagnostic audiologic assessment, 0.5 percent were confirmed to have hearing loss.

Universal Newborn Screening

As a result of concerns about the long-term developmental implications of delayed identification, evaluation, and treatment of hearing loss in children, Congress authorized the development of a system of early hearing detection and intervention programs. By 2005, all states had operational programs. The programs seek to identify congenital, permanent bilateral or unilateral sensory, or permanent conductive hearing loss and neural hearing loss. Children are initially screened in the hospital using physiological techniques (automated auditory brainstem responses or otoacoustic emissions). Those who were born outside of a hospital or who missed or failed the initial screen are screened/rescreened by 1 month of age. Those who do not pass the rescreening are referred for audiologic evaluation by 3 months and, if they are found to have a hearing loss, referred for aural rehabilitation, medical, and early intervention services by 6 months of age.

Initial screening has proved to be very successful. The Centers for Disease Control and Prevention (CDC) reported that in 2007, approximately 95 percent of eligible infants were screened by early hearing and intervention programs. However, a significant number of children who required further evaluation did not receive appropriate follow-up evaluations. Of the 1.8 percent of children who did not pass their initial screen, 37 percent were found to have normal hearing, and 6.3 percent of children who failed the screen had a hearing loss. Unfortunately,

56.6 percent of children who failed the initial screen did not have a documented diagnosis. Of this group, 79 percent were either lost to follow-up or lost to documentation, 13 percent were in process, and the remainder had parents who declined further evaluation or moved to another state, or the child died.

Of the children with hearing loss, 85.5 percent were referred for early intervention services (Part C of IDEA). Of concern was that 35.7 percent of children with hearing loss were not receiving early intervention, the vast majority of whom were lost to follow-up/documentation.

The AAP Joint Committee on Infant Hearing (2007) identified a number of challenges to the success of the Early Hearing Detection and Intervention (EHDI) systems. Among them were (1) too many children were lost between the failed screening and rescreening and between the failed rescreening and the diagnostic evaluation, (2) often there is a lack of timely referral for diagnosis of and intervention for suspected hearing loss in children, (3) access to Part C services is inadequate among states and within states, (4) there is a lack of specialized services for children with multiple disabilities and hearing loss, and (5) there is a shortage of professionals with skills and expertise in both pediatrics and hearing loss and a lack of in-service education for key professionals. Early childhood personnel can play an important role in assuring that children who fail a screen receive the necessary evaluation to confirm or exclude the diagnosis of hearing impairment.

WHAT ARE THE LIMITS OF EARLY IDENTIFICATION?

Early identification is part of a process that leads to early intervention and better outcomes for the individual. Systems for identifying developmental disabilities have improved significantly over the past quarter century, but still there are limits to achieving the goals of early identification of all children with developmental disabilities. Among the factors that limit early identification efforts are the need to have multiple evaluations to detect all of the disorders of interest, the limited ability of current instruments to classify children successfully, and insufficient efforts to ensure that children who are identified with early identification techniques receive confirmatory testing and, ultimately, intervention.

Early identification does not take place at a single time. It is not possible to identify all possible conditions of interest at a single time.

Sometimes time must pass before the symptoms of a disorder show themselves well enough to be identified. Our current instruments for identification are limited in their ability to identify children with developmental disabilities. Consequently, children may have to "grow into" a disorder. Identification of developmental disabilities is a continuing process. Recognition of this led the AAP to develop a system that includes ongoing surveillance and screening at multiple ages (AAP Committee on Children with Disabilities et al., 2006).

Early identification does not always result in early intervention. The Early Hearing Detection and Intervention Program is a model for identification, but it is limited. Systems that bridge identification and intervention programs are often inefficient. Families may be difficult to follow or may not appreciate the potential of early intervention. Again, early childhood personnel can be key advocates to assure that children receive the follow-up evaluations and, when necessary, referrals for services that they need.

The costs of early identification programs are not trivial. Among the costs are contacting and gaining permission for screening, informing those who fail the screening tests and ensuring that they receive confirmatory screening, provision of counseling relative to the disorder of interest, and linking to early intervention services. Decisions must be made by policy makers as to how much to expend in early identification and how much to allow for other programs.

Early identification is not independent of the other processes that affect the outcome of individuals with developmental disabilities. While it focuses on the individual, early identification is dependent on processes that affect the community and family environments. Unless it is coupled with research that focuses on better techniques for identification, improved methods of intervention, increased understanding of the roles of families in identification and intervention, and successful ways of preventing developmental disabilities, early identification will not meet its objectives.

References

Allen, R. L., Stuart, A., Everett, D., & Elangovan, S. (2004). Preschool hearing screening: Pass/refer rates for children enrolled in a head start program in eastern North Carolina. *American Journal of Audiology, 13*(1), 29–38.

American Academy of Pediatrics Committee on Practice and Ambulatory Medicine of American Academy of Pediatrics, Section on Ophthalmology of American Academy of Pediatrics, American Association of Certified Orthoptists, American

Association for Pediatric Ophthalmology and Strabismus, and American Academy of Ophthalmology. (2003). Eye examination in infants, children, and young adults by pediatricians. *Pediatrics, 111,* 902–907.

American Academy of Pediatrics Council on Children with Disabilities, Section on Developmental Behavioral Pediatrics, Bright Futures Steering Committee, Medical Home Initiatives for Children with Special Needs Project Advisory. (2006). Identifying infants and young children with developmental disorders in the medical home: an algorithm for developmental surveillance and screening. *Pediatrics, 118*(1), 405–420.

American Academy of Pediatrics Joint Committee on Infant Hearing. (2007). Year 2007 position statement: Principles and guidelines for early hearing detection and intervention programs. *Pediatrics, 120*(4), 898–921.

American Speech-Language-Hearing Association (ASHA). (1997). Guidelines for audiologic screening. Retrieved December 17, 2010, from http://www.asha.org/docs/html/GL1997-00199.html doi:10.1044/policy.GL1997-00199

Bruer, J. T. (1999). *The myth of the first three years.* New York: The Free Press.

Centers for Disease Control and Prevention. Summary of 2007 National EHDI Data (Version 1). Retrieved December 17, 2010, from http://www.cdc.gov/ncbddd/ehdi/documents/DataSource2007.pdf

Centers for Disease Control and Prevention. http://www.cdc.gov/ncbddd/dd/default.htm

Committee on Practice and Ambulatory Medicine, Section on Ophthalmology, American Association of Certified Orthoptists; American Association for Pediatric Ophthalmology and Strabismus; American Academy of Ophthalmology. (2003). Eye examination in infants, children, and young adults by pediatricians. *Pediatrics, 111*(4, pt. 1), 902–907.

Gesell, A., & Amatruda, C. S. (1947). *Developmental diagnosis* (2nd ed.). New York: Hoeber.

Hartmann, E. E., Bradford, G. E., Chaplin, P. K., Johnson, T., Kemper, A. R., Kim, S., & Marsh-Tootle, W. (2006). PUPVS panel for the American Academy of Pediatrics. Project. Universal Preschool Vision Screening: A demonstration project. *Pediatrics, 117*(2), 226–237.

Lock, T. M., Shapiro, B. K., Ross, & Capute A. J. (1986). Age of presentation in developmental disability. *Journal of Developmental and Behavioral Pediatrics, 7*(6), 340–345.

McCormick, D. P., Johnson, D. L., & Baldwin, C. D. (2006). Early middle ear effusion and school achievement at age seven years. *Ambulatory Pediatrics, 6*(5), 280–287.

Nance, W. E. (2003) The genetics of deafness. *Mental Retardation Developmental Disabilities: Research Reviews, 9*(2), 109–119.

National Research Council and Institute of Medicine. (2000). From neurons to neighborhoods: The science of early child development. In J. P. Shonkoff & D. A. Phillips (Eds.), *Board on Children, Youth, and Families, Commission on Behavioral and Social Science and Education.* Washington, DC: National Academy Press.

Paradise, J. L., Campbell, T. F., Dollaghan, C. A., Feldman, H. M., Bernard, B. S., Colborn, D. K., et al. (2005). Developmental outcomes after early or delayed insertion of tympanostomy tubes. *New England Journal of Medicine, 353*(6), 576–586.

P.L. 106-402. (2000). Developmental Disabilities Assistance and Bill of Rights Act of 2000. 114 stat.1683–1684.

P.L. 108-446. (2004). Individuals with Disabilities Education Act of 2004. 118 Stat 2657–2658.

Pulsifer, M. B., Hoon, A. H., Palmer, F. B., Gopalan R., & Capute, A. J. (1994). Maternal estimates of developmental age in preschool children. *Journal of Pediatrics, 125*(1), S18–24.

Roizen, N. J. (2003). Nongenetic causes of hearing loss. *Mental Retardation Developmental Disabilities: Research Reviews, 9*(2), 120–127.

Shapiro, B. K., & Gwynn, H. (2008). Neurodevelopmental assessment of infants and young children. In A. J. Capute & J. A. Accardo (Eds.) *Neurodevelopmental disabilities in infancy and childhood.* Baltimore: Paul H. Brookes.

State of Maryland Family Health Administration. Newborn Blood Spot Screening Program. http://fha.maryland.gov/genetics/nbs_bloodspot.cfm

Tingley, D. H. (2007). Vision screening essentials: Screening today for eye disorders in the pediatric patient. *Pediatrics in Review, 28,* 54–61.

Chapter 5

Professional Development for Early Childhood Intervention: Current Status and Future Directions

Susan A. Fowler, Tweety Yates, and Michaelene M. Ostrosky

P rofessional preparation is a central issue in early childhood education, with many hotly debated questions at the core of this issue. For example, what constitutes a highly qualified teacher or provider who can serve all young children, including those with special needs (e.g., developmental delays) or those at risk for later school difficulties (e.g., living in poverty, English-language learners)? What professional preparation should early childhood educators receive *before* they work with young children? Should their preparation include a college degree, license, certificate, credential, or endorsement? What ongoing professional development would benefit early childhood educators *after* they begin working with young children and families? Across the United States, these questions are not easily or consistently answered. The philosophy that young children with special needs and their families are full members of their community, and that they should receive services in their natural environments or in programs that serve typically developing children, is an important piece of any discussion of personnel preparation. However, the issue of *who* provides *what* services for young children and *where* these services are provided is complex for several reasons.

First, the personnel who work with young children during the early years (before kindergarten) come from many different disciplines and begin their careers in early education with varying levels of preparation. Whether personnel are licensed, credentialed, or meet minimum training requirements depend on a variety of factors, including place of employment, services provided, characteristics of the children served, state regulations, and even sources of funding. Their titles and training vary by position (teacher, aide, therapist, provider, early interventionist) as well as by specialization (e.g., developmental therapist, speech therapist, early childhood special education teacher, infant toddler specialist, child care provider). Their preparation may or may not have included a focus on working with young children with special needs or diverse abilities.

Second, the number of children who enter group care or receive care outside of the home has increased dramatically in the past few decades, as more parents are involved in the workforce. This has placed a great demand on the need for personnel in early care and education, making it one of the fastest-growing sectors in the workforce (Bartsch, 2009). National surveys currently estimate that over 11 million children receive some form of early care and education outside of the home annually during their first five years of life (Burton et al., 2002). To meet this need, an estimated 2.2 million individuals are paid annually to provide care and education to society's youngest members (Brandon, Weiss, & Dugger, 2010).

Third, there is no single service system or model for meeting the educational, therapeutic, or child care needs of young children below the age of 5. Instead we have a variety of services that include publicly funded programs, such as Head Start, state funded prekindergarten, and early childhood special education, as well as private programs (for profit and not for profit), such as nursery schools and part-day and full-day child care. Some programs are licensed by a state regulatory agency, and others are licensed exempt. Some programs are located in community settings (e.g., park districts), while others reside in religious settings (e.g., churches), corporate settings, or local school districts. In total, half of the early care and education teachers and staff (1.1 million) work within center-based contexts. Family child care is yet another source of care, which may be provided for a fee or through less formal avenues such as kith and kin systems of exchange. Family child care likewise can be licensed or unlicensed, and annually, 300,000 individuals provide family child care (care for small groups of children who are not related and receive service in the provider's home). Yet another option used by many families is paid relatives and non-relatives who provide care; of these, an estimated 600,000 are relatives and 200,000 are non-relatives or neighbors (Brandon et al., 2010). The level of preparation and formal training for early care and education providers varies greatly, especially given the setting. Those who work in regulated settings, such as community-based centers, tend to have the greatest level of education and may hold licenses, certificates, or credentials. Each state sets its own licensing standards and regulates child care training. Requirements may range from less than a high school diploma to college degree. Thus, *where* personnel work and *what* they do in their work also dictates their level of preparation (U.S. Department of Labor, Bureau of Labor Statistics, 2010).

PERSONNEL WHO PROVIDE SPECIAL EDUCATION AND RELATED SERVICES TO YOUNG CHILDREN

It is within this larger context of early care and education that services for children with developmental delays and disabilities must be considered. The number of children identified as eligible for early intervention (birth to age 3) and early childhood special education (ages 3–5) services has doubled over the past 20 years since all states were required to provide services to all eligible preschool-aged children and to have a system of early intervention in place for infants and toddlers. Recent federal data indicate that over one million children received special education and related services during their first five years. In 2008, 710,000 children between the ages of 3 and kindergarten entry were served through early childhood special education services. Approximately 322,000 infants and toddlers with developmental delays received early intervention services during their first three years of life (USDE 28th Annual Report to Congress, 2009), and increasingly, many children with disabilities or developmental delays receive early care and education services alongside their typically developing peers. In fact, 2006 data indicate that approximately one-third of preschool-aged children with disabilities receive all of their special education and related services in typical early childhood settings, and an additional 17 percent of children attend a typical early childhood program at least part of the time while also attending a specialized program. Figure 5.1 presents the distribution of educational environments where 3- to 5-year-olds received special education and related services in 2006. The most recent reauthorization of the Individuals with Education Improvement Act (2004) emphasized the importance of educating children with disabilities in the same settings in which their typically developing peers are educated. As a result, the percentage of children with disabilities who are enrolled in programs that also serve typically developing children is likely to increase even more.

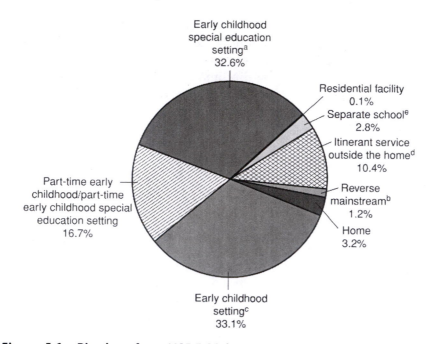

Figure 5.1   Pie chart from USDE 28th Annual Report to Congress (Figure 1-13; distribution of educational environments where children ages 3 through 5 are receiving special education and related services under IDEA, Part B: Fall 2004, p. 35).

The location of services for the very youngest children, newborns through age 2, have also been addressed through policy and statute, which require that services be delivered in natural environments, defined as settings in which children without disabilities are most likely to be served. In many instances, the natural environment is the home, and services are provided through home visits or in community locations requested by the family. This is a shift away from the delivery of services in clinical or medical settings or in programs designed solely for children with disabilities. It is also a shift toward providing intervention in the context of a family's daily routine, so that families or other caregivers are likely to participate in the intervention and apply the strategies or practices throughout typical daily activities.

With these demographic and contextual variables in mind, the purpose of this chapter is to discuss the current state of professional preparation for the array of personnel who work directly with very young children (birth to age 5) who have developmental delays or disabilities and with their families. The focus of the chapter is primarily on those who are certified, licensed, or credentialed to work with children with special needs. However some attention is given to personnel who have not been prepared to work with children with disabilities, but who play a central role in their care and education in community programs.

EARLY INTERVENTION SERVICES FOR INFANTS AND TODDLERS AND THEIR FAMILIES (EI)

The goal of Early Intervention (EI) is to provide support to infants, toddlers, and young children and their primary caregivers to promote optimal development during the first three years of life. An essential philosophical element of EI is to strengthen and support the parents' or caregivers' capacity to meet their child's needs and design services within the context of the family (Dunst, 2007). To optimize state resources, the original legislation (EHA, 1986) identified the basic components that should be included in EI systems, while allowing states the flexibility of determining the population served as well as the structure of their service delivery system. Given this flexibility, *how* services are provided as well as *who* provides these services can vary greatly from state to state (Bruder, 2010). Table 5.1 presents the professional fields originally identified within early intervention. Current research indicates that the most commonly provided services are: special instruction and child development, speech therapy, occupational therapy, physical therapy, developmental therapy, and service coordination (Hebbeler, Spiker, Morrison, & Mallik, 2008).

Table 5.1   Disciplines Identified by PL 99-457 as Eligible Providers of Services for Infants and Toddlers with Exceptionalities and Their Families

Audiology

Medicine

Nursing

Nutrition

Occupational Therapy

Physical Therapy

Psychology

Special Education

Speech Therapy

Social Work

Development of Early Intervention Credential and Preparation Systems

The original 1986 legislation gave states a five-year window to develop a coordinated and comprehensive infrastructure for providing early intervention services. Two components of this system included the development of personnel standards and a comprehensive system of personnel development (CSPD) that included both preservice and in-service preparation of personnel (McCollum & Bailey, 1991). While most states already had professional preparation standards and state licensure for teachers in early childhood special education, the majority did not have standards or credentials for providers serving infants and toddlers. Many states saw the opportunity for the development of an early intervention credential as a way to improve the quality of their EI services and personnel development systems. The credential would provide a method for a state-identified entity to review providers' experiences and qualifications related to serving very young children as well as ensure an understanding of the EI system. A primary question became *how* to create a credentialing system that encompassed multiple disciplines from different training programs, with varying licensure requirements and philosophies for delivering services (Bruder, Mogro-Wilson, Stayton, & Dietrich, 2009; Campbell, Sawyer, & Muhlenhaupt, 2009).

Despite these challenges, recent reports indicate that approximately half of the states either have or are developing a credential specific to early intervention (the Center to Inform Personnel Preparation Policy and Practice in Early Intervention and Preschool Education, 2007). The primary method for obtaining a credential in early intervention involves meeting competency standards (as developed by individual states). The credential attests that personnel have demonstrated competencies related to working with infants and toddlers with disabilities and their families. These standards may be met by attending in-service trainings, completing coursework, or through a recognized program of preservice preparation. An example of South Carolina's core competencies for early intervention providers can be found in Table 5.2. The core competencies are listed as well as one example of a required skill under each competency area.

Many states have added systems overview trainings as a prerequisite before personnel could begin providing services. These trainings typically include an overview of the state philosophy and principles around early intervention and legal requirements of early intervention.

Table 5.2   Sample Competencies in EI

South Carolina Early Intervention Core Competencies (http://www.scfirststeps.org/
BabyNet/Policies%20and%20Procedures/Appendix7d.pdf)

1. Early Intervention Foundations

Example: Know and apply relevant policies and procedures regarding the
components of a Part C system: Interagency collaboration, public awareness and
child find, referral and intake, evaluation, assessment and determination of
eligibility, IFSP development, implementation, and monitoring transition, service
coordination training, teaming, and consultation, and procedural safeguards, due
process, and mediation.

2. Child Development and Learning

Example: Understand typical and atypical child development and the implications
for development and learning.

3. Family and Community Relationships and Supports

Example: Establish and maintain collaborative partnerships with families that build
families' sense of parenting competence and confidence.

4. Evaluation and Assessment

Example: Use a variety of screening, evaluation, and assessment methods and
tools in a family-centered and culturally sensitive manner.

5. Service Coordination, Delivery, and Implementation

Example: Implement and monitor an Individualized Family Service Plan (IFSP) that
incorporates child and family outcomes within the context of the family's home
and community routines and activities.

6. Professional Development Standards

Example: Incorporate current scientifically based research findings/trends and
peer-reviewed literature relevant to early intervention systems and services to
solve problems and/or modify existing practices with families, infants, and toddlers.

Trainings may also include information on the operation of the system
(e.g., billing procedures for services, processes for family referral and
evaluation). Another major training focus is how early intervention is
conducted between families and professionals within natural environments. Professional development efforts increasingly have focused on
providing services in natural environments using a family-centered
philosophy and a transdisciplinary approach (Bruder, Mogro-Wilsom,
Stayton, & Dietrich, 2009; Campbell, Sawyer, & Muhlenhaupt, 2009).

Traditionally, early intervention had been viewed as child-focused,
with the major purpose being to enhance the developmental outcomes
for young children with disabilities. This shift in practice was based

primarily on two interrelated reasons: the child is a member of the family, and the family has significant impact on the child's development. Thus, the primary role of service providers in EI became to work with and support family members and caregivers in children's lives. In addition, a new emphasis was placed on providing EI services in natural environments as defined by individual states. This change resulted from research showing that it is during routine activities and everyday interactions with familiar people in familiar contexts that learning opportunities occur for children. In addition, special instruction by early interventionists seemed to be most effective within the context of natural environments using a team approach among professionals and parents (Dunst, 2007). This shift to providing services in natural environments presented not only a change in where services were provided but also a change in how they were provided. A set of guiding principles was developed to illustrate these beliefs and how these practices should support intervention with all children and families within natural environments. These principles can be found in Table 5.3 (NECTAC Workgroup on Principles and Practices in Natural Environments, 2008).

Use of natural environments represents a significant philosophical shift in service orientation for those specialists whose preparation may

Table 5.3   NECTAC Work Group Principles and Practices for Providing Early Intervention in Natural Environments (2008)

Seven Principles for Providing Early Intervention in Natural Environments

1. Infants and toddlers learn best through everyday experiences and interactions with familiar people in familiar contexts.
2. All families, with the necessary supports and resources, can enhance their children's learning and development.
3. The primary role of the service provider in early intervention is to work with and support the family members and caregivers in a child's life.
4. The early intervention process, from initial contacts through transition, must be dynamic and individualized to reflect the child's and family members' preferences, learning styles, and cultural beliefs.
5. IFSP outcomes must be functional and based on children's and families' needs and priorities.
6. The family's priorities, needs, and interests are addressed most appropriately by a primary provider who represents and receives team and community support.
7. Interventions with young children and family members must be based on explicit principles, validated practices, best available research, and relevant laws and regulations.

have focused on the delivery of services to older children or even adults in school, clinical, and medical settings. In fact, a recent study of service delivery combinations in early intervention found that when children received services from multiple therapists, the therapists were "less likely to provide services in the home only and more likely to offer a combination of group and one-on-one. Furthermore, these families were most likely to receive the highest intensity of services per week (i.e, more than 2 hours)" (Raspa, Hebbeler, Bailey, & Scarborough, 2010, p. 140–141). This finding was also true with speech therapist services. This study identified the five most typical teams of providers who worked with families in EI. The five teams included (1) speech language pathologist, (2) occupational-physical therapist, (3) educator team, (4) multiple-therapist team, and (5) other provider teams. They found that the educator team and the occupational-physical therapist teams were most likely to provide services one-on-one and in the home (Raspa, Hebbeler, Bailey, &Scarborough, 2010). The majority of states have established EI technical assistance systems to support the training of providers. Many states are relying on in-service development to provide additional training to specialists to prepare them for the specific concerns and issues of meeting the needs of very young children and their families through natural environments.

A Growing Profession

A shortage of personnel in many of the identified disciplines has further exacerbated state efforts to develop and support their credentialing systems and professional development plans. States reported shortages of speech therapists, occupational therapists, physical therapists, and special educators. As a way to address personnel shortages, about half of the states reported adding new professional categories, particularly at the paraprofessional level including speech language therapist assistants, physical therapist assistants, and occupational therapist assistants. In addition, several states reported adding professional parent roles such as parent facilitators and parent liaisons. Other states added bilingual and sign-language interpreters, not only to improve the number and quality of EI personnel, but also to meet the growing need for more diverse and culturally competent staff.

While there is no question that much progress has been made as states have put systems into place to ensure that EI providers have the knowledge, skills, and abilities to work with infants and toddlers with disabilities and their families, there are still several important issues to be addressed. Among these are the different ways in which states fund services for families and their young children. A number of states have moved to a system of fee-for-service, in which individual therapists or providers are reimbursed for the time that they spend working directly with a family. Although their services may be coordinated through a local office, they work as independent contractors. This means that supervision is minimal and the opportunity to participate in reimbursed professional development is missing (Peterson, Luze, Eshbaugh, Jeon, & Kantz, 2007). Fee-for-service structures also may interfere with the opportunity for providers to meet and engage in transdisciplinary planning and the development of interventions that can address multiple areas of growth and development for the family and reduce the number of providers in their lives.

Challenges for EI Personnel

First, while many states have developed credentialing systems and training requirements, few have created an avenue or career ladder for early intervention providers to advance within the system based on training and performance. This would not only strengthen the quality of services provided in the system, but also help in retaining quality personnel. Secondly, with the ongoing challenge of personnel shortages, states will need to determine how to maintain their standards of excellence while meeting the increased need for additional personnel. Lastly, support is needed to increase the number of higher-education programs and qualified faculty offering EI coursework. Results from the Center to Inform Personnel Preparation Policy and Practice in Early Intervention and Preschool Education (2005) showed that while only a little over half of the states reported having higher education programs that prepared professionals to work in the field of EI.

EARLY CHILDHOOD SPECIAL EDUCATION (ECSE): SERVICES FOR CHILDREN FROM BIRTH TO AGE 8

While Early Intervention is defined as a service field for children from birth through age 2, the age range of children served within early childhood education and early childhood special education can vary considerably based on state definitions. As in Early Intervention, personnel from several disciplines are involved in the delivery of services to preschool-aged children with disabilities. These include early childhood special educators (ECSE), early childhood educators (ECE), paraprofessionals, speech and language therapists, occupational therapists, physical therapists, and other related services (e.g., nursing, nutrition). Shortages have been reported in most of these disciplines for serving preschool-aged children (Center to Support Personnel Preparation and Practice, 2007). This section of the chapter will address the role of ECSE and ECE teachers and their current status. In general, early childhood special education refers to free, appropriate, specially designed instruction to meet the unique needs of a young child with a disability. Common to all states with some form of ECSE preparation program is the delivery of services to children between three years of age and the age of eligibility for kindergarten. The instruction and services can be delivered in a preschool classroom, in the home, in child care, or in other settings in which preschool-aged children typically are found (http://www.isbe.state.il.us/earlychi/pdf/ECSE_LRE_guidance.pdf). The majority of children with disabilities between the ages of 3 and 5 are served in classroom settings, with only 3 percent receiving services at home (Carlson, et al., 2008; Markowitz et al., 2006; USDE 28th Annual Report to Congress, 2009). However, many states may provide certification or endorsements in ECSE that allow educators to work with children across a variety of age ranges (e.g., birth to age 8, age 3 to 21). Certification is acquired through the completion of a baccalaureate degree or an advanced degree. Endorsements are considered as add-on requirements beyond the initial certification, which expand the range of children a teacher may serve. The variability in age ranges across states, as well as the use of endorsements and certifications, creates a complicated context for the preparation of personnel who seek to work primarily with young children.

The need for personnel in ECSE increased dramatically 25 years ago when federal legislation and funding expanded services to all children between ages 3 and 5 who were identified as having a disability or developmental delay. Prior legislation had permitted services for younger children but had not required them. As a result, over half of the states did not have services in place for all preschool-aged children with disabilities; and of these, many did not have teacher preparation programs or certification requirements for early childhood special education. Most states had requirements in place for special education (often crossing the age range of 3–21) and for early childhood education (ECE), but not for the intersection of the two professions. The need to certify a sufficient pool of ECSE teachers quickly outpaced efforts to develop policies that might create a uniform certificate for all teachers in early childhood, whether special education or general education. The early requirement for meeting the least restrictive environment for serving children with disabilities allowed for (1) locating classes for preschool children with disabilities in regular elementary schools; (2) linking classes for children with disabilities part time with other public programs, such as Head Start; and (3) placing children with disabilities in private community programs (USDE Federal Register, 1989). This initial flexibility with which service could be provided resulted in many school districts adding self-contained classes in neighborhood elementary schools, although the second and third options also were used, but with less frequency.

With the increased demand for ECSE teachers, new personnel preparation programs were developed across the country; some emerged from special education programs, others from early childhood education programs, and a few from a blending of the two programs. Currently, 80 percent of the states require an ECSE certificate to teach preschool-aged children with disabilities, in the role of either co-teacher, consultant, itinerant, or primary teacher (Geiger, Crutchfield, & Mainzer, 2003). The route to certification, however, can vary considerably from state to state, as can the age ranges served through the certification. Although teachers are required to be certified to teach preschoolers with disabilities, the most recent federal report on certification indicates that as many as 12 percent of teachers employed to provide special education and related services to preschoolers are not fully certified (USDE 28th Annual Report to Congress, 2009).

In an effort to create greater uniformity and consistency in preparation programs, the major association for early childhood education, the National Association for the Education of Young Children (NAEYC), and the primary association for early childhood special education, the Division of Early Childhood of the Council of Exceptional Children (DEC), both recommended that states develop free-standing certificates for professionals who work with young children from birth through 8 years of age. Their statements advocate that professionals be certified for the same age ranges and that states adopt the same standards for certification to increase reciprocity (Hyson, 2003; Sandell, McLean, & Smith, 2000).

A basic element of their shared approach is the delineation of three age ranges for children who are taught within ECE and ECSE: infants and toddlers (birth through age 2), preschool (ages 3 to 5 or kindergarten entry), and primary (kindergarten to third grade). The statement recommends that certification programs allow personnel to choose specializations in two of the three age spans. Such specialization supports the idea that personnel should gain the knowledge and skills most appropriate for promoting learning and development in very young children (birth to age 5) or children entering their early years of education (ages 3 to 8). This recommendation that all states support a congruent age range for certification is intended not only to increase reciprocity among states, but also to create a uniform and distinctive certificate that addresses the skills and knowledge around assessments, curriculum, and teaching strategies needed for supporting young children.

A review of state certification requirements for ECSE teachers indicates that states are far from meeting the ideals of shared certification standards and consistent age ranges. A recent study of requirements indicates that six certification models are used across the country (Stayton et al., 2009) and that at least 11 age ranges are represented across these models within the United States.

Models of Certification for Early Childhood Special Education

Table 5.4 reflects the emerging nature of ECSE as a specialized content area and the extent to which it may be most closely associated with special education, early childhood education, or both. As such, some states have certification in ECSE, and others have endorsements in ECSE. The distinctions impact the model of preparation. States with ECSE certification have adopted a set of regulated requirements that prepare teachers to work specifically with young children who have disabilities or developmental delays. States with the ECSE endorsement, in contrast, have teachers complete a set of requirements that are added to an existing teaching certificate, which could be early childhood education

Table 5.4   Models of Certification for Early Childhood Special Education

1. ECSE certification
2. ECSE endorsement
3. Blended ECE and ECSE certification
4. Special education certification
5. ECSE and special education endorsement
6. ECE and special education endorsement

or special education. Endorsements are "add-ons" to a program and typically involve additional coursework and practice teaching. The extent to which endorsement programs actually integrate information on teaching children with and without disabilities into the same coursework, or present them as separate courses, varies.

The blended ECE and ECSE certification ideally is a program that prepares teachers to work with typically developing children as well as those with disabilities, and addresses the range of child abilities throughout shared coursework and field experiences. This is the model that approximates the joint position statement on inclusion developed by DEC and NAEYC and enables teachers to work in classrooms that are inclusive of all children. The blended certificate also allows teachers the flexibility to teach within the general education system or special education system. It supports the inclusion of children with disabilities with typically developing peers. A teacher with the blended certification may be the primary teacher or co-teacher within an inclusive early care and education program, or serve as a consultant to a number of programs that include children with disabilities. They might also teach in an inclusive class in elementary schools, such as first grade. Interviews with state directors of ECSE services identified three themes behind the development of the blended certificate. The first was to provide inclusion opportunities for children, the second was to enhance collaboration between general and special education in teaching children, and the third was to increase the professional status of early childhood and early childhood special educators in the field (Stayton et al., 2009).

The fourth model, special education certificate, reflects an extension of teacher preparation in special education to include preschoolers along with students enrolled in kindergarten through grade 12. Some states have a special education certificate that covers the full range of children with disabilities from age 3 to age 18 or 21. Teachers prepared in these programs may subsequently teach a variety of age groups and are less likely to have much coursework and experience with young children. The fifth and sixth models identified are ones in which teachers have a certificate but hold multiple endorsements, whether in special education or in early childhood. Interestingly, some states follow a single certification route, while others use several of the models as pathways for teachers to become certified. This may reflect a need for flexibility in hiring personnel for programs as well as the patchwork pattern in which routes to certification or endorsement have developed over time.

The core content of preparation programs is another way in which the national associations are working toward consensus and a shared approach to accreditation of college and university preparation programs. The Council of Exceptional Children (CEC), which is the parent organization of DEC, has identified 10 common core standards that all special educators must meet. DEC has added six standards specific to ECSE preparation in addition to the core standards (Council for Exceptional Children, 2009). If a higher education program offers a blended ECE and ECSE degree, then NAEYC standards also are included in the program. Table 5.5 presents the standards developed by CEC for all special education teachers, the DEC standards added specifically for early childhood special education, and the NAEYC standards for early childhood care and education. The standards share a focus on (1) promoting child learning, (2) linking child assessment with teaching or instruction, and (3) professional development. Collaboration is clearly identified in CEC and DEC as an important standard representing the need to build relationships with professionals in related specialties (e.g., speech therapy) and in general education for the inclusion of students. This standard also includes collaboration with families, which likewise is emphasized in several of the NAEYC standards.

In a recent study, 17 states were sampled to determine if state early childhood special education standards were congruent with nationally recommended standards. Again, the variability across states in meeting the standards was striking. Three of the 17 states met or nearly met all ECSE standards and the CEC common core, while another two states met more than half of the standards. These five states indicated that they either adopted the national standards or aligned their state standards directly with the national standards. In contrast, three states met none of the standards, and the remaining nine ranged from meeting slightly more than 10 percent to fewer than 50 percent. (Center to Inform Personnel Preparation Policy and Practice in Early Intervention & Preschool Education, 2008). This lack of convergence between state and national standards indicates that most states are working in isolation in developing and revising their certification requirements. Many do not appear prepared or able to adopt nationally advocated standards. In fact, interviews conducted with state policy makers suggest that experts in ECSE may not even be at the table for discussion of certification and endorsement standards related to early childhood education. One policy maker was quoted as saying, "certification development and implementation is a slow, cumbersome process in

Table 5.5   Standards for Professional Development in Special Education, Early Childhood Special Education, and Early Childhood Education

Council for Exceptional Children: Core Standards for All Special Educators	Division for Early Childhood of CEC: Standards for ECSE	National Association for the Education of Young Children: Standards for ECE
1. Foundations	1. Leadership and policy	1. Promoting child development and learning
2. Development and characteristics of learners	2. Program development and organization	2. Building family and community relationships
3. Individual learning differences	3. Research and Inquiry	3. Observing, documenting and assessing to support young children and families
4. Instructional strategies	4. Individual and program evaluation	4. Using developmentally effective approaches to connect with children and families
5. Learning environments and social interaction	5. Professional development and ethical practice	5. Using content knowledge to build meaningful curriculum
6. Language	6. Collaboration	6. Becoming a professional
7. Instructional planning		
8. Assessment		
9. Professional and ethical practice		
10. Collaboration		

Source: CEC, 2009; NAEYC, 2009

which key stakeholders in the state with expertise in ECSE may not be integrally involved in the process" (p. 11). This is in direct contrast to the national associations' recommendation that personnel standards be developed within a collaborative framework including representation of key stakeholders and representatives of professional organizations, policy makers, and families. Given the small percentage of state certification efforts that align with national standards, most states may take years to reach the ideals established by the national professional associations. The lack of alignment between states, and with national standards, will continue to create barriers to reciprocity of certifications and endorsements for highly qualified teachers, making it impractical to recruit across state lines. Nonetheless, national organizations continue to advocate for more consistency in philosophy and approach.

Inclusive Early Childhood Programs

The blended model of ECE and ECSE, or the ability for teachers to have an endorsement in one area and certification in the other, will increase in popularity and demand due to other educational changes in the nation. In 2004, the Individuals with Disabilities Education Act was reauthorized and included language that explicitly stated that young children with disabilities were to be served in the same settings that children without disabilities are served. This clarification of the least restrictive environment option for children, preschool and school aged, has increased significantly the percentage of children who are served in the general education environment with access to the general education curriculum. The U.S. Department of Education reported in 2009 that half of preschool-aged children were enrolled either full time or part time in early childhood settings (USDE 28th Annual Report to Congress, 2009).

Perhaps just as important as the legislative direction was the development and adoption in 2009 by DEC and NAEYC of their first joint position statement entitled *Early Childhood Inclusion* (see Tables 5.5 and 5.6). The organizations noted:

> [T]he lack of a shared national definition has contributed to misunderstandings about inclusion ... and that having a common understanding ... is fundamentally important for determining what types of practices and supports are necessary to achieve high-quality inclusion. (DEC/NAEYC, 2009, p. 1)

The publication of this statement places even more pressure on states to create professional development programs so that all teachers have the skills and competencies to work with all children, including those with and without disabilities. In fact, the organizations call for a revision of program and professional standards, stating: "A definition of inclusion could be used as the basis for revising programs and

Table 5.6 Definition of Early Childhood Inclusion from the DEC/ NAEYC Joint Position Statement on Inclusion

Early childhood inclusion embodies the values, policies, and practices that support the right of every infant and young child and his or her family, regardless of ability, to participate in a broad range of activities and contexts as full members of families, communities, and society. The desired results of inclusive experiences for children with and without disabilities and their families include a sense of belonging and membership, positive social relationships and friendships, and development and learning to reach their full potential. The defining features of inclusion that can be used to identify high-quality early childhood programs and services are access, participation, and supports.

professional standards to incorporate high-quality inclusive practices" (p. 4). Likewise, it also calls for "an integrated system of high-quality professional development to support the inclusion of young children with and without disabilities" (p. 4). The joint statement on inclusion has the potential to push states to develop both preservice, in-service, and technical assistance programs that will prepare early childhood educators to work with all children.

The emergence of the pre-K or universal preschool movement in the last decade also has increased opportunities for the inclusion of children with IEPs, providing a more normalized or natural environment for children with disabilities. As of 2010, 38 states provide publicly funded pre-K services for 3- and 4-year-olds. In fact, the 2009 Report on "The State of Preschool" in the United States indicates that "30 percent of children attend a state-funded preschool program at age 4, including those receiving special education. When Head Start is added, enrollment in public programs is nearly 40 percent at age 4" (Barnett, Epstein, Friedman, Sansanelli, & Huestedt, 2009, p. 1). As a result, many states and their local districts are including children with IEPs in their pre-K classes using a model in which ECSE and ECE teachers team-teach, or in which an ECSE teacher oversees the implementation of the IEP by consulting with the ECE teacher, who is the lead teacher for the classroom. This is a dramatic shift from the use of self-contained ECSE classes in neighborhood schools, initially allowed in 1988.

Recent research has focused on identifying the factors likely to influence the successful inclusion of children with disabilities in community preschool programs designed for typically developing children or children at risk due to poverty. Access to ongoing professional development has been identified as a key factor (Lieber et al., 2000). One study of 16 preschool programs across four states found that training was critical for staff to address the particular needs of a child with disabilities as well as to include the child in typical activities, whether by adapting materials or using supports, such as a peer or staff member. Another study identified limited qualified personnel as a barrier to inclusion (Brotherson, Sherriff, Milburn, & Schertz, 2001). Not surprisingly other issues that influenced successful inclusion included the opportunity for staff to have time to plan and coordinate services, the development of respectful relationships among the early care and education teachers, and the specialized therapists and teachers. Having a shared vision for inclusion and the transformations in classrooms and teacher roles to support inclusion likewise is often cited (e.g., Buysee, Wesley, & Keyes, 1998).

Because inclusive child care and education is not universally available for all families with a young child with a disability, many have to put together two or more programs to meet their child's special education needs as well as the family's need for child care. Their children make a daily transition between a half-day ECSE program designed to meet their special needs and a child care. These transitions may range from simple and almost seamless to difficult to negotiate, depending on the child and the relationships between program staff and family. For example, if there are no links between home, preschool, and child care, then only the child knows what happens in each setting and may or may not be able to convey critical events. Programs that have regularly scheduled communication (such as notebooks that travel, phone calls, and e-mail) can improve the quality and consistency of services that children receive and at the very least keep each other and the family well informed about each day. Research on the extent to and ways in which teachers communicate across programs for children who are dually enrolled is limited. But one research study indicates that several barriers can impact sharing of information. They range from time constraints and logistics of communication to attitudes in which teachers report lack of willingness or respect on the part of one program. Interestingly, communication was most likely to occur in response to a child's behavior problems in one program and the desire to identify a common and effective way of intervening or circumventing the undesirable behaviors (Donegan, Ostrosky, & Fowler, 1996). Again, joint in-service training opportunities could address issues of attitude and respect by providing opportunities for ECSE teachers and ECE and child care providers to learn about ways of collaborating and ways of supporting the child and family in the two programs and addressing specific strengths and needs.

INCREASED DEMAND FOR CERTIFIED ECE TEACHERS

The increase in publicly funded prekindergarten programs, the recent expansion of Head Start services, and the professionalization of its teaching force are among several factors that are leading to increased professionalization of early care and education teachers—those teachers who work outside of the public school sector. Most early childhood teachers who are not certified have at least an associate of arts degree (Kagan, Kauerz, & Tarrant, 2008). Teachers who hold the title of lead teacher typically have more education than assistant teachers. Teachers in state-funded prekindergarten programs or those certified to work with preschool children with disabilities tend to be the most educated, holding baccalaureate or graduate degrees and certifications. Increased education, along with employment in state or federally funded preschool programs, has led to significantly higher salaries for teachers, with ECSE teachers and certified ECE teachers in public pre-K programs being paid at school-district salary levels. According to the U.S. Department of Labor, National Bureau of Labor Statistics (2007), salary figures nationally averaged $51,160 for ECSE teachers. In contrast, licensed or certified preschool teachers who work outside of pre-K programs were likely to earn half as much, or $25,800. Those who were employed as child care providers were likely to earn even less, averaging $19,670. Preschool teachers earn less than any other teacher in the field of education, and child care workers are among the lowest paid in the service care industry. The degree to which economic and educational improvements in one sector of early care and education improve the conditions for other sectors is yet unknown. However, the knowledge and skills of teachers in early care and education are important factors to consider, as children with disabilities are increasingly spending all or part of their day in early care and education programs, where their peers without disabilities are served. Significant disparities in pay and status among teachers who hold certification and those who do not may also impact their successful collaboration in community programs (Fink & Fowler, 1997). Conversely, the higher status and salary of certified teachers may lead to changes in the status of noncertified teachers and promote a focus on a career ladder within the field that will enable teachers to move toward higher credentials or certification based on continued professional development and ultimately to more competitive salaries.

THE FUTURE OF EI/ECSE PROFESSIONALS

The fields of EI/ECSE continue to evolve, developing primarily in the past 25 years. Empirical research has shown that high-quality early childhood programs for infants, toddlers, and preschoolers result in positive outcomes for children as well as later success in school and the community (Raver, 2002). Early childhood is recognized as the critical period for brain development; this time in young children's lives establishes the foundations of language development, social and emotional development, and a predisposition to learning and curiosity. Standards and benchmarks for early child learning and development have been established in states throughout the country. Teacher preparation standards have been proposed by international and national organizations (i.e., DEC, NAEYC, Head Start) and licensures, certifications, and credentials have been developed to ensure quality early childhood programming and to advance professionalism in an area that has not been traditionally valued by society at large (as evidenced by low salaries in child care and high turnover rates). Even with these improvements in standards and professionalism, the fields of ECSE and EI still face challenges, including shortages. For instance, the numbers of professionals and paraprofessionals who provide early intervention services for infants, toddlers, and young children number around 63,000, and the number of teachers with ECSE endorsements and/or certifications number near 31,000 (USDE 28th Annual Report to Congress, 2009). States have developed a greater capacity to serve young children and their families, and they have improved their processes for identifying eligible children. Over the past 20 years, the number of children receiving services has doubled to more than a million.

Concurrent with the changes in early intervention and special education have been dramatic changes in the population of young children born in the United States. Advances in medical technology have enabled more very low-birth-weight, premature infants to survive, many of whom will require early intervention services. The demographic changes in the child population are dramatic, with 20 percent of all children living in homes with at least one immigrant parent, with many children speaking a first language other than English.

In contrast, most teachers and providers in early care and education are likely to be white, female, and in their 30s or 40s. Greater diversity in terms of race and ethnicity can be found in programs in which at least 75 percent of the children are from an underrepresented group. However, there is a significant ethnic, racial, gender, and linguistic gap between the increasingly diverse population of children and the primarily white, female, and English-speaking professionals who serve young children (Saluja, Early, & Clifford, 2002). This mismatch in demographics can be problematic as the diversity of the early childhood population is not represented in the adults who teach and care for them. Acknowledging and celebrating families' cultures, home languages, and values are critical when creating partnerships and facilitating young children's development and learning. Cultural clashes are more likely to occur when those who teach our youngest members of society have backgrounds that are different from the families of those in their care. Misunderstanding may arise around family and professional roles, child-rearing practices, and cultural traditions and values. For example, a common myth held by many educators is that children should learn one language at a time and that speaking multiple languages will confuse or delay young children's acquisition of English (Tabor, 2008). Yet, globally, most people are multilingual. Cultural competence and an appreciation of multilingual homes must be part of the awareness and skill set of all beginning and practicing early educators. The extent to which cultural and linguistic diversity is addressed in depth in preparation programs is very uneven (Sanchez & Thorpe, 2008) Professional preparation programs, whether preservice or in-service will need to address the changing demographics and infuse diversity constructs into all aspects of early education (Maude et al., 2010).

Another topic receiving considerable attention in special education is the use of scientifically based or evidence-based practices (EBP), which has emerged from the medical field. With the introduction of No Child Left Behind legislation, the U.S. Department of Education began emphasizing the importance of considering the research evidence behind intervention strategies and instructional practices (Buysee & Wesley, 2006). As the fields of general and special education struggle to define EBPs (and what type of information counts as evidence for good practice), a second hurdle facing the fields is to prepare and support teachers in implementing EBPs. Translating research to practice cannot be achieved without close attention to the fidelity with which any particular practice is implemented by professionals

(Odom, 2009). If we believe that EBPs and high-quality teachers are linked, then professional development must include an emphasis on defining, implementing, and evaluating EBPs.

The current emphasis on EBP is impacting the field of early childhood special education as teachers are pushed to critically evaluate the evidence behind the practices they consider embracing. Administrators also are challenged to provide teachers with the time, tools (i.e., coaching and mentoring in using a practice correctly), and resources (i.e., access to professional journals, involvement in research projects) necessary to implement evidence-based practices. Professional organizations (e.g., Division of Early Childhood of the Council for Exceptional Children) and Web sites (e.g., the What Works Clearinghouse) are excellent resources for learning about EBPs in early childhood special education.

Technology may represent another challenge and area of growth for personnel in EI and ECSE. As new technologies emerge, early interventionists and early childhood special education professionals should be encouraged (and expected) to master these tools as they would other tools of their trade. The ways we communicate, access information, and connect with one another are changing. Young adults often turn first to technology for obtaining new information and for networking with peers and other professionals (e.g., the Internet, Facebook, Twitter, and mobile devices that provide access to many resources and offer opportunity for collaborative work). Young families may turn first to Web resources for advice and information and find competing recommendations or explanations for their questions. Helping families to navigate resources may become another part of the job for EI providers and early childhood teachers.

Technology also has implications for the preparation of future teachers and therapists. Researchers have already begun investigating the use of technology to provide immediate feedback to student interns (Barton & Wolery, 2007) and to provide consultative support when implementing interventions (Gibson, Pennington, Stenhoff, & Hopper, 2010). In fact, technology may provide part of the solution to preparing more teachers and in supporting advancement on the career ladder as online classes and distance education provide access to continuing education for a broad range of individuals.

Retaining new teachers and therapists in their positions can be as much of a challenge as preparing a sufficient supply. One strategy is to provide mentoring and induction to novice teachers, including those in EI and ECSE. Smith and Ingersoll (2004) note that new teacher induction programs are "designed to assist novice teachers to move from their role as a pre-service 'student of teaching' to their new role as a 'teacher of students' " (p. 683). Induction programs may include "workshops, collaborations, support systems, orientation seminars, and especially mentoring" (Smith & Ingersoll, 2004, p. 683). Although induction has been discussed in the teacher education literature for many years (Feiman-Nemser, Schwille, Carver, & Yusko, 1999; Wong, 2004), attention to the design and implementation of meaningful induction activities for novice teachers is critical at this time when U.S. public schools are faced with growing demands to recruit and prepare teachers to address the needs of an increasingly diverse student population.

Keeping teachers employed at the same school or in the same early childhood program (as well as keeping early interventionists employed in their role, such as independent developmental therapists) provides stability for students and their families and reduces costs for schools and communities. Teacher stability is especially problematic for the field of special education. Darling-Hammond and colleagues (2005) describe four factors that influence the retention of new teachers: (1) salaries, (2) working conditions, (3) preparation, and (4) mentoring support.

As the fields of EI and ECSE move out of the infancy stage, high-quality preservice training, professional development, opportunities for planning and collaborating with peers, the availability of mentoring and induction programs, and other such resources are necessary. They are critical to increasing the diversity of the professionals who enter the field and in preparing them to work with and meet the unique needs of our youngest members of society and their families. Those who provide professional preparation to future generations of early childhood educators must continue to refine and improve pre-service and in-service offerings so the most current information, reflecting evidence-based practices, is available to practitioners. Early interventionists and early childhood special educators who provide an array of services to infants, toddlers, and young children with and without disabilities in a variety of settings deserve nothing less than the best preparation and support available so that they in turn can provide the optimal services to young children and their families.

References

Barnett, W. S., Epstein, D. J., Friedman, A. H., Sansanelli, R. A., & Huestedt, J. T. (2009). *The state of preschool 2009*. National Institute for Early Education Research. Retrieved from http://nieer.org/yearbook

Barton, E. E., & Wolery, M. (2007). Evaluation of email feedback on the verbal behaviors of pre-service teachers. *Journal of Early Intervention, 30*(1), 55–72.

Bartsch, J. S. (2009) The employment projections for 2008–18. *Monthly Labor Review Online, 132*, No. 11. Retrieved from http://www.bls.gov/opub/mlr/2009/11/art1exc.htm

Brandon, R. N., Weiss, E., & Dugger, R. (2010). The economic value of U.S. early childhood investments. Presented at the NACCRRA Policy Symposium, Washington, DC. Retrieved from http://www.naccrra.org/conferences/symposium/docs/The%20Economic%20Value%20of%20Early%20Childhood%20in%20the%20US.pdf

Brotherson, M., Sherriff, G., Milbrun, P., & Schertz, M. (2001). Elementary school principals and their needs and issues for inclusive early childhood programs. *Topics in Early Childhood Special Education, 21,* 31–45.

Bruder, M. B. (2000). Family centered early intervention: Clarifying our values for the new millennium. *Topics in Early Childhood Special Education, 20*(2), 105–115.

Bruder, M. B. (2010). Early childhood intervention: A promise to children and their families for their future. *Exceptional Children, 76,* 339–355.

Bruder, M. B., Mogro-Wilson, C., Stayton, V., & Dietrich, S. L. (2009). The national status of in-service professional development systems for early intervention and early childhood special education practitioners. *Infants and Young Children, 22,* 13–20.

Burton, A., Whitebrook, M., Young, M., Bellm, D., Wayne, C., & Brandon, R. N. (2002). *Estimating the size and components of the U.S. childcare workforce and caregiving population: Key findings from the child care workforce estimate.* Washington, DC: Center for the Child Care Workforce and Human Services Policy Center.

Buysee, V., & Wesley, P. W. (2006) Evidence-based practice: How did it emerge and what does it really mean for the early childhood field? In V. Buysee & P. W. Wesley (Eds.), *Evidence-based practice in the early childhood field.* Washington, DC: Zero to Three.

Buysse, V., Wesley, P., & Keyes, L. (1998). Implementing early childhood inclusion: Barrier and support factors. *Early Childhood Research Quarterly, 13,* 169–184.

Carlson, E., Daley, T., Bitterman, A., Riley, J., Keller, B., Jenkins, F., & Markowitz, J. (2008). *Changes in the characteristics, services, and performance of preschoolers with disabilities from 2003–04 to 2004–05, wave 2 overview report from the pre-elementary education longitudinal study.* Rockville, MD: Westat. Retrieved from https://www.peels.org/reports.asp

Campbell, P. H., Sawyer, L. B., & Muhlenhaupt, M. (2009). The meaning of natural environments for parents and professionals. *Infants and Young Children, 22,* 213–224.

Center to Inform Personnel Preparation Policy and Practice in Early Intervention & Preschool Education. (2005). Study II data report: The higher education survey for early intervention and early childhood special education—Preparing adequate numbers of students in institutions of higher education trained in service areas required under the IDEA. Retrieved from http://www.uconnucedd.org/projects/per_prep/per_prep_resources.html

Center to Inform Personnel Preparation Policy and Practice in Early Intervention & Preschool Education. (2006). *Study IV data report: The national status of early intervention personnel credentials*. Retrieved from http://www.uconnucedd.org/projects/per_prep/per_prep_resources.html

Center to Inform Personnel Preparation Policy and Practice in Early Intervention & Preschool Education. (2007). Study 1, The national landscape of early intervention in personnel preparation standards under Part C of the Individuals with Disabilities Education Act (IDEA), Vol. 1. Retrieved from http://www.uconnucedd.org/projects/per_prep/per_prep_resources.html

Center to Inform Personnel Preparation Policy and Practice in Early Intervention & Preschool Education. (2008). Study V Data Report: Analysis of State Certification Requirements for Early Childhood Special Educators. Retrieved from http://www.uconnucedd.org/projects/per_prep/resources/LP-revision12-11-Study V FINAL Data Report with Content Analysis 01-23-09 ccs.pdf

Council for Exceptional Children. (2009). *What every special educator must know ethics, standards and guidelines* (6th ed.). Arlington, VA: Author.

Darling-Hammond, L., Holtzman, D., Gatlin, S. J., & Heilig, J. V. (2005). Does teacher preparation matter? Evidence about teacher certification, Teach for America, and teacher effectiveness. *Education Policy Analysis Archives, 13*(42). Retrieved from http://epaa.asu.edu/epaa/v13n42

DEC/NAEYC. (2009). Early childhood inclusion: A joint position statement of the Division for Early Childhood (DEC) and the National Association for the Education of Young Children (NAEYC). *Young Exceptional Children, 12,* 42–47.

Donegan, M. M., Ostrosky, M. M., & Fowler, S. A. (1996). Children enrolled in multiple programs: Characteristics, supports and barriers to teacher communication. *Journal of Early Intervention, 20,* 95–106.

Dunst, C. J. (2007). Early intervention for infants and toddlers with developmental disabilities. In S. L. Odom, R. H. Horner, M. E. Snell, & J. Blatcher (Eds.), *Handbook of developmental disabilities* (pp. 161–180). New York: Guilford Press.

Feiman-Nemser, S., Schwille, S., Carver, C., & Yusko, B. (1999). *A conceptual review of literature on new teacher induction*. Washington, DC: National Partnership for Excellence and Accountability in Teaching.

Fink, D. B., & Fowler, S. A. (1997). Inclusion, one step at a time: A case study of communication and decision making across program boundaries. *Topics in Early Childhood Special Education, 17*(3), 337–362.

Geiger, W. L., Crutchfield, M. D., & Mainzer, R. (2003). The status of licensure of special education teachers in the 21st century. Retrieved from http://www.copsse.org

Gibson, J. L., Pennington, R. C., Stenhoff, D. M., & Hopper, J. S. (2010). Using desktop videoconferencing to deliver interventions to a preschool student with autism. *Topics in Early Childhood Special Education, 29*(4), 214–225.

Hebbeler, K. Spiker, D., Morrison, K., & Mallik, S. (2008). A national look at the characteristics of Part C early intervention services. In C. A. Peterson, L. Fox, & P. M. Blasco (Eds.), *Young Exceptional Children Monograph Series No. 10: Early intervention for infants and toddlers and their families: Practices and outcomes* (pp. 1–18). Longmont, CO: Sopris West.

Hyson, M. (2003). *Preparing early childhood professionals: NAEYC's standards for programs*. Washington, DC: National Association for the Education of Young Children.

Illinois State Board of Education. (2005, September). Early childhood special education least restrictive environment (LRE) guidance paper. Retrieved from http://www.isbe.state.il.us/earlychi/pdf/ECSE_LRE_guidance.pdf

Individuals with Disabilities Education Improvement Act Amendments of 2004, Pub, L. No. 108-446, 118 Stat. 2647 Retrieved from http://www.copyright.gov/legislation/pl108-446.pdf

Kagan, S. L., Kaurez, K., & Tarrant, K. (2008). *The early care and education teaching workforce at the fulcrum: An agenda for reform.* New York: Teachers College Press.

Lieber, J., Hanson, M., Beckman, P., Odom, S., Sandall, S., Schwartz, I., et al. (2000). Key influences on the initiation and implementation of inclusive preschool programs. *Exceptional Children, 67,* 83–98.

Markowitz, J., Carlson, E., Frey, W., Riley, J., Shimshak, A., Heinzen, H., et al. (2006). *Preschoolers' characteristics, services, and results: Wave 1 overview report from the pre-elementary education longitudinal study (PEELS).* Rockville, MD: Westat. Retrieved from https://www.peels.org/reports.asp

Maude, S. P., Catlett, C., Moore, S., Sanchez, S. Y., Thorp, E. K., & Corso, R. (2010) Infusing diversity constructs in preservice teacher preparation: The impact of a systematic faculty development strategy. *Infants and Young Children, 23,* 103–121.

McCollum, J., & Bailey, D. (1991). Developing comprehensive personnel systems: Issues and alternatives. *Journal of Early Intervention, 12*(3), 195–211.

National Association for the Education of Young Children (NAEYC). Standards for professional preparation programs. (2009). Retrieved from http://www.naeyc.org/positionstatements/ppp

NECTAC Work Group on Principles and Practices in Natural Environments. (2008). Agreed upon practices for providing services in Natural Environments. Retrieved from http://www.nectac.org/~pdfs/topics/families/AgreedUponPractices_FinalDraft2_01_08.pdf

Odom, S. L. (2009). The tie that binds: Evidence-based practice, implementation science, and outcomes for children. *Topics in Early Childhood Special Education, 29*(1), 53–61.

Peterson, C. A., Luze, G. J., Eshbaugh, E., Jeon, H. J., & Kantz, K. R. (2007). Effecting change through home visiting: Promising pathways or unfulfilled expectations. *Journal of Early Intervention, 29,* 119–140.

Raspa, M., Hebbeler, K., Bailey, D. B., & Scarborough, A. A. (2010). Service provider combinations and the delivery of early intervention services to children and families. *Infants & Young Children, 23*(2), 132–144.

Raver, C. (2002). Emotions matter: Making the case for the role of young children's emotional development for early school readiness. *Social Policy Report, Society for Research in Child Development, 16,* 3–20.

Saluja, G., Early, D. M., & Clifford, R. M. (2002). Demographic characteristics of early childhood teachers and structural elements of early care and education in the United States. *Early Childhood Research and Practice, 4,* 285–306.

Sanchez, S., & Thorpe, E. (2008). Teaching to transform: Infusing cultural and linguistic diversity. In P. J. Winton, J. A., McCollum, & C. Catlett (Eds.), *Practical approaches to early childhood professional development: Evidence, strategies, and resources* (pp. 81–97). Washington, DC: Zero to Three.

Sandall, S., McLean, M. E., & Smith, B. J. (Eds.). (2000). *DEC recommended practices in early intervention/early childhood special education* (pp. 1–168). Longmont, CO: Sopris West.

Smith, T. M., & Ingersoll, R. M. (2004). What are the effects of induction and mentoring on beginning teacher turnover? *American Educational Research Journal, 41* (3), 681–714.

Stayton, V. D., Dietrich, S. L., Smith, B. J., Bruder, M. B., Mogro-Wilson, C., & Swigart, A. (2009). State certification requirements for early childhood special educators. *Infants and Young Children, 22,* 4–12.

Tabor, P. (2008). *One child: Two languages: A guide for early childhood educators of children learning English as a second language* (2nd ed.). Baltimore: Brookes Publishing Company.

Wong, H. K. (2004). Induction programs that keep new teachers teaching and improving. *National Association of Secondary School Principals (NASSP) Bulletin, 88*(638), 41–58.

U.S. Department of Education, *Federal Register.* (1989, April 27). 34 CFR Part 300, Assistance to states for education of handicapped children; final regulations (pp. 18254–18255). Washington, DC: U.S. Government Printing Office.

U.S. Department of Education, 28th annual report to Congress on the implementation of the Individuals with Disabilities Education Act, 2006. (2009). Retrieved from http://www2.ed.gov/about/reports/annual/osep/2006/parts-b-c/index.html

U.S. Department of Labor, National Bureau of Labor Statistics. (2007–08). *Occupational outlook handbook2010–2011 Edition*: Child care workers. Retrieved from http://www/bls.gov/oco/ocos170.htm

What Works Clearinghouse. Retrieved from http://ies.ed.gov/ncee/wwc

Chapter 6

Trends in Contemporary American Families and Their Significance for Young Children

Bahira Sherif Trask and Steven Eidelman

From a practice, research, and policy perspective, families play a crucial role in American children's lives. For children with disabilities, this is even more true. Many of the systems of services and supports, especially Part C of the Individuals with Disabilities Education Act (IDEA) and Head Start programs have strong family components. For children with significant disabilities, there is frequently more interaction with the health care system, further placing additional responsibilities on families.

Recent surveys indicate that, despite media portrayals to the contrary, most Americans still place a high value on finding a significant other, marrying for love, and having children (Saad, 2006). Historically, families were formed through marriage. Marriage marked the formation of a new household, the initiation of a sexual relationship, and the birth of children. With the increasing social acceptance of premarital sex, cohabitation, childbirth outside of marriage, and same-sex partnerships, fundamental notions about who or what is a family are increasingly debated. The institution of family is being redefined. These debates around the public and private roles of families have brought to the forefront a series of policy concerns, many of which center specifically on improving the welfare of children and their development. Moreover, contemporary discourses around families increasingly acknowledge the critical role that other structures and institutions in society play. These discourses have served to highlight the fact that "family" can be experienced differently by children depending on their social class, race, ethnicity, gender, disabilities, and even regional location.

The current financial downturn has highlighted the realization that although some families and their children are more vulnerable than others to economic marginalization, none are immune from the deep structural changes undermining "traditional" families. Contemporary adaptation in families has taken varying forms including renegotiated gender roles, increasing divorce rates, the increase in single-parent households, and more nonfamilial household units. Moreover, as social and economic changes produce new family arrangements, some of these alternatives are becoming more accepted, in the face of rhetoric to the contrary. Rather than being an expression of group-specific differences alone, family diversity is an outgrowth of distinctive patterns in the way families and their members are embedded in environments with varying access to opportunities, resources, and rewards.

THE MYTH OF THE MONOLITHIC FAMILY

The term "the family" has become increasingly controversial over the last several decades. It is associated with a specific composition of members and their associated roles. To most Americans, the term "family" conjures up an image of a father, mother, and children, with the father gainfully employed and the mother, ideally, a homemaker available to her children at all times. Critics argue that most individuals in U.S. society do not live in that arrangement anymore, and that, thus, the term "the family" has lost its functional meaning. Later in this chapter, data are presented related to this point. For these critics, the concept of the family is also problematic because it is understood to be prescriptive (i.e., it implies how people *should* live and does not reflect the reality of most Americans' lives). Smith (1993) has referred to this as the Standard North American Family (SNAF), and maintains that this image is still powerful even though the realities for most American families are quite different. According to the U.S. Census Bureau (2008), approximately 7 percent of households in the United States consist of a father gainfully employed in the labor force, a mother who is a homemaker, and their children. If divorce and remarriage were factored in, the percentage of families who fit this particular family type would be even smaller.

Currently, the legal definition of family, used by the U.S. Census Bureau, refers to two or more people who live together in a household and are related to each other by blood, marriage, or adoption. This definition of families is structural; it focuses on the requirements for membership and the spatial arrangements (where they are living together or in separate physical locations) of its members. In 2007, there were 116 million U.S. households. Of those, approximately, 67.8 percent (78.4 million) of all households fit this U.S. Census Bureau definition of family. This statistic indicates a decrease in family households from 85 percent in 1960, which can be attributed to various factors including: individuals are marrying later, they are less likely to have children, and they are more likely to live alone or with an unrelated person. The number of households composed of married couples with children under the age of 18 dropped from 40 percent in 1970 to 23 percent in 2007, while the number of individuals living alone doubled from 13.1 percent to 26.8 percent. Male-headed households with a child or other dependent family member jumped from 2.4 percent in 1960 to 4.4 percent in 2007. Female-headed households with a child or dependent family member climbed from 8.4 percent to 12.4 percent (U.S. Census Bureau, 2008), an increase of nearly 50 percent. There has also been an increase in the number of nonfamily households that contain more than one individual, more than doubling from 1.9 percent to 5.6 percent. This number may conceal gay or heterosexual couples who are living together without being formally married as well as renters or boarders in homes. These statistics indicate that while married households are still in the majority, an increasing number of young and old individuals are living in arrangements that are not officially defined as family, though the people in these arrangements may consider themselves to be in a family.

While household composition has changed, so has the average size of families and households. In 2007, the average American household is estimated to have about 2.56 individuals. This figure represents a significant reduction when compared to some of the earliest census figures. Census figures from 1890 indicate that the average American household at that time contained 5.4 individuals, more than double the average size of today's households.

Statistics on households and families, however, are deceptive. Families are not just defined by their structures. Most Americans now consider any group of emotionally bonded individuals as a family (Stacey, 1996). Families are linked to societal ideologies and reflect certain values and behaviors that are considered important in a culture. Understanding these behaviors and values is critical because they provide an explanation for why certain types of families are legitimized. They also set the criteria for what is considered deviant. Social arrangements that are considered deviant are not supported through public opinion or through social policies. This occurs to maintain a specific type of social order. For example, over the last several years, we have witnessed strident debates around same-sex marriage in the United States. While same-sex marriage is legitimized by law in many European countries, we in the United States have been slow to accept the formal union of gay and lesbian couples. The debates over same-sex marriage provide an example of the relative power of different interest groups—in this case, heterosexual versus homosexual individuals. These disputes also give us insight into the fundamental values that many Americans still hold when it comes to the institution of family—that families are created through marriage between a man and a woman.

Despite controversies around the definition and meaning of family, families in the United States continue to enjoy significant symbolic value. Politicians run for office emphasizing their strong "family values." Commercial ventures such as the Disney Channel promote "family programming," implying that they are geared toward promoting the psychological health and well-being of children. Countless other products and services are marketed as being "family friendly." Much of this symbolism implies that families are wholesome units, united with respect to goals, and sharing uniform experiences. These idealized versions of family life have been challenged in particular by feminists, who have revealed that the internal workings of families are not necessarily in line with public representations. For example, Heidi Hartmann introduced the idea that families are often wrought with conflict and represent conflicting interests.

> Such a view assumes the unity of interests among family members: it stresses the role of the family as a unit and tends to downplay conflicts or differences of interest among family members. I offer an alternative concept of the family as a locus of struggles. In my view, the family cannot be understood solely or even primarily as a unit shaped by affection or kinship, but must be seen as a location where production and redistribution take place. As such, it is a location where people with different activities and interests in these processes often come into conflict with one another. (Hartmann, 1981, p. 368)

Hartmann's perspective highlighted the notion that families are places where individuals negotiate their different relationships and desires. Different members will have varied perspectives on their experiences in their families. Thus, some members may feel that their families are "happy families" though other members may feel quite negatively about their experiences within the same family. This perspective allows us to understand that the internal dynamics of families are often quite different depending on the vantage point of different individuals. Different children may have very diverse experiences within the same family, depending on birth order, gender, disabilities, and a myriad of other factors.

CHANGES IN AMERICAN FAMILIES

Much of the contemporary controversy around families centers on perceived or suspected transformations in American families. However, what is often not clearly understood is that much of the change with respect to families is actually the result of demographic transformations, and not necessarily just the consequence of family dissolution and family intimacy, as is so often believed (Fischer & Hout, 2010). For example, one major change over the last 100 years is that Americans are living longer. In 1900, an American white male was expected to live until approximately the age of 62 or 63. Today, an American white male can expect to live until his mid-70s, and the estimates for middle- and upper-class males is quite a bit higher. The same facts hold true for women. This greater longevity has significant implications for family life and for social policies pertaining to families. Children today are much more likely to know their grandparents, and even their great-grandparents, than at any other time in human history (Buck, Van Wel, Knijn, & Hagendoorn, 2008). However, the greater longevity of family members has also introduced significant concerns around caretaking responsibilities for adult children, and at times even for younger children and children with disabilities, in families (Bengston & Allen, 1993). Many families raising young children are also providing care to aged parents.

Moreover, another demographic shift, the declining fertility of women, has had a profound impact on families. While in 1900 the average American woman bore about four children, today's mother averages about two children (with some differences between different ethnic and religious groups). These extensions of the life span and the reduced fertility of women have contributed to a large number of Americans over 50 living in the "empty nest" with just a spouse, and an increasing number of older individuals living alone (Fischer &

Hout, 2010). Thus, the most profound change in contemporary American family life has been experienced by the elderly, who are the most likely to have ended their parenting at an earlier stage in life, have fewer children, and are living longer than past generations.

Another profound family change in the United States centers around the large proportion of mothers with young children now working in the paid labor force. In 1920, approximately 10 percent of married women worked outside of the home. In 2008, 60 percent of mothers with preschool children were employed outside of the home, with the rate for low-income women higher than for middle-class women. This trend has significant implications for the raising of children, the relationship between spouses, and for community and social life. Mothers have more pressure on their time, are significantly responsible for child care arrangements, and are still expected to perform household duties (U.S. Department of Labor, 2009, Table 7).

Families who have a child with a significant disability are more likely to be poor and more likely to experience material hardship than families without a child with a disability (Parish et. al., 2009). These same families, with higher costs for raising their child (or children) with disabilities, are also more likely to work fewer hours due to care-giving burdens, though the evidence for this is not as strong as the cost of caregiving evidence, and therefore have fewer financial resources available to them (Rupp & Ressler, 2009).

Other significant family trends include the rising age of marriage for both women and men and the continued high divorce rate. The age of first marriage has fluctuated somewhat over the last 100 years, with a dip in marriage age occurring in the 1950s but rising steadily to about 25 years for women and 28 years for men in 2009 (U.S. Census Bureau, 2009). With respect to divorce, it is important to note that, historically, marriages were more likely to be dissolved through the death of a spouse than through the legal termination of a marriage. Today, while divorce has become commonplace, so has remarriage and cohabitation. As will be discussed later, there is a great deal of academic and popular dispute around the effects of divorce on children; however, in reality, we know little about the processes of divorce on the development of children when coupled with remarriage and periods of cohabitation.

There has been a great deal of misinformation about the divorce rate in families where there is a child with a disability. The research demonstrates mixed impacts, with some studies showing a higher divorce rate when there is a child who was born with low birth weight, cerebral palsy (Joesch & Smith, 1997), attention deficit hyperactivity disorder (ADHD), and oppositional defiant disorder (Wymbs et. al., 2008), though the impact is not high. Other studies on children with intellectual disability or children with autism do not show a significant difference, though a lot has been written about stress on the family and emotional stress on the parents (Bromley, Hare, Davison, & Emerson, 2004; Yamada et al., 2007). While beyond the scope of this chapter, the impact of a child on families is something early childhood providers should be aware of in their work.

Interestingly, marriage remains as popular an option as always in the United States. When polled, over 90 percent of Americans claim that they want to marry—and actually do marry (Fischer & Hout, 2010). From an historical perspective, it is actually simpler to create a stable nuclear family for children in the contemporary context because premature death and unplanned pregnancies, while still over 40 percent of all pregnancies, have become less common.

A BRIEF OVERVIEW OF HISTORICAL ASPECTS OF AMERICAN FAMILIES

The transition from subsistence farming to wage labor that began in the late 1700s marked the origins of many of the trends witnessed in today's American families. As commercial capitalism with its emphasis on the buying, selling, and distribution of goods such as tobacco, grain, and cotton took hold, new types of jobs became available that drew men, primarily sons, off their family farms and undermined the authority of fathers. As children attained a greater degree of economic independence, they were also able to subscribe to more individualistic notions of family life. By the mid-1800s, as industrial capitalism spread, increased factory work had changed the nature of both work and family life.

In agrarian times, women and men worked together to maintain the farm and the household. Then, industrialization moved work out of the home. The industrial form of wage labor became increasingly valued as society moved predominantly toward a market economy (Hattery, 2001). The movement toward industrialization was accompanied by a growing distinction between men's (paid) work and women's (unpaid) work. As the need for factory labor grew, men's work became more valuable and led to a societal belief in the "natural" roles of men and women. This pervasive belief in a "natural" division of labor became legitimized by emphasizing the biological differences between the sexes. Women's biological ability to bear children became equated with an equivalently important ability to rear children. Among the American middle and upper class, this was thought to make women more suited to attending to the private sphere of the household and family. Men, on the other hand, were believed to be biologically better disposed to working in the harsh environments of factories and, in general, in the public arenas of work and finance. This economic transformation created a context in which the contributions of men came to be perceived as more valuable for families and society due to the primacy given to the importance of earning money (Moen & Sweet, 2003). Women's most important input became their domestic one. Feminists have pointed out that by working for "free," women's labor became undervalued, creating inequalities in families. These eighteenth- and nineteenth-century developments gave birth to an ideology about gender roles and the division of labor in families that continues to persist in U.S. culture.

Contemporary feminist scholarship on families has exposed this inequality between the sexes in families and questioned the arrangement of "traditional" families with respect to the roles of women (Hattery, 2001). In much of this literature, family arrangements that foster the well-being of children have been virtually ignored. Instead, the primary emphasis in much of the research on families has continued to focus on issues around the perpetuation of traditional models of gender. Despite a lack of interest specifically in children, much of this work has revealed that popular conceptualizations of historically stable, breadwinner-homemaker families with happy, well-adjusted children has no real foundation in reality! Instead, historically, most American families were not able to adhere to a model of family life with two parents who were biologically related to their children, clear gender roles, and a father employed in the labor force. Instead, death often left children without one or both parents, and poverty often forced all members of the family, including the children, to work to survive. For low-income, immigrant, and minority men and women, family constellations that deviated from the mainstream ideal were the norm, not the exception. In these families, women most commonly worked outside of the home to help make ends meet, and men and children shared in domestic household activities including caretaking (Coontz, 1992).

From an historical perspective, there were several other noteworthy developments in American families that continue to play a role in contemporary social life. Throughout much of American history, love and sex were not a significant aspect of marriage and the founding of families. In fact, until about 1900, passion was thought to be a dangerous emotion that should not be part of the marriage process. Instead, parents played a critical role in helping choose a mate for their children. Criteria for marriage included a suitable family background, economics, sympathy, and understanding. Men and women married for economic reasons, social stability, social acceptance, and to have children (Cherlin, 2010).

Between 1890 and 1960, attitudes towards families, marriage, and sex underwent a profound transformation. Increasingly during this period, sexual attraction and love came to be seen as the most important criteria in choosing a mate. Individuals no longer married just to produce children anymore. Moreover, with the introduction of birth control and better health practices, childhood mortality sank, and men and women were able to have fewer children. The life span of family members also increased. The shift toward smaller families that were living longer allowed men and women to focus their attention on each other and to emphasize the psycho-social development of their children.

Changes within families were also accompanied by new attitudes toward children. In colonial times, children were to have been born "in sin" and were, thus, raised very strictly. It was only in the late 1800s that attitudes toward children began to shift. Children were now believed to be morally pure and closer to God than adults, which led to a new way of viewing parenting. Children were now consigned to the "women's sphere" as they were believed to need their mother's nurturance and guidance. This was, again, a significant shift in family life. During colonial times, men had been believed to be the better, more appropriate parent and spiritual guide of their children. It is important to note that these conceptualizations of the purity and innocence of children were reserved again, however, for white middle-class children. African American, working-class, and immigrant children were expected to work and assume adult roles from a very early age. They did not participate in the new conceptualizations of children as moral and pure, worthy of a labor- and worry-free childhood.

The 1960s introduced new social perspectives on families that had their roots in the civil rights movement, the expansion of sexual behavior outside of marriage, the Vietnam War, the revival of feminism, and a general anti-authoritarian stance. The divorce rate started to climb to unprecedented rates, and women with children flocked into the work force. While statistics indicate an increase in the percentage of two-parent families during the decades of the 1950s, 1960s, and 1970s (Seward, 1978), Masnick and Bane (1980) point out that it was only in the late 1970s that the number of nuclear families affected by divorce began to exceed those disrupted by death. As the prevalence of divorce and mothers with children under age 18 entering the work force increased, American families began to deviate from the 1950s and 1960s concept of the "typical" or "traditional" family. The general shift away from the family as a unit of production to a unit characterized by emotional intimacy is today seen by many scholars as the primary transformation in American family life (Coontz, 1992).

In the late twentieth and early twenty-first centuries, other notable family trends have accompanied ideological changes. Fertility has decreased while cohabitation has increased, and "other" forms of families such as step-families, female-headed households, and grandparents raising children have become increasingly visible. In particular, gay and lesbian families have become a recognized, if controversial, family form in Western families. Nevertheless, research indicates that gay and lesbian couples look for the same things that other men and women search for in their relationships: commitment, stability, and companionship as well as satisfying sexual relationships. Gay and lesbian couples, however, tend to be more egalitarian than heterosexual couples. Gay and lesbian families share similar goals and expectations for family life. Many individuals and couples are choosing to become parents; however, current legislation preventing legal marriage and same-sex adoptions in many states present unique challenges to family formation (see http://gaylife.about.com/od/gayparentingadop tion/a/gaycoupleadopt.htm). Regardless of the legal obstacles that face many gay and lesbian couples, a sociological phenomenon labeled the "gayby boom" has led to significant number of same-sex partners and gay and lesbian individuals choosing to have children and providing a supportive and healthy environment for child rearing. Currently, approximately one in three lesbian women has given birth to a child, and one in six gay men has either adopted or fathered a child (Gates, Badgett, Macomber, & Chambers, 2007). It is important to acknowledge, however, that gay and lesbian families continue to face discrimination despite the growing number of individuals and families advocating for social equity regardless of sexual orientation.

THE FAMILY VALUES DEBATE

The contemporary trend of high numbers of women working outside of the home has set the stage for an unprecedented degree of debate about the appropriate distribution of roles in families. From an historical perspective, in the United States until the early 1960s, most women who sought employment outside of the home were poor and women of color. White women participated in the labor force only during their early 20s, leaving once they married and had children. A short deviation from this pattern occurred during World War II, when women were needed in the labor force due to a shortage of men. However, with the return of large numbers of men from the military after World War II, women were encouraged to once again take up their domestic roles. Beginning in the late 1960s, a new trend emerged: women entered into the labor force and remained through their childbearing years (Bianchi, Robinson, & Milkie, 2007).

In the United States, the debate about women's and men's roles has taken on strong political connotations. It is primarily referred to as the "family values" debate even though, in reality, it focuses on women's paid employment and the resultant changes in family life. For example, one prominent scholar has suggested that "families have lost functions, power, and authority; that familism as a cultural value has diminished, and that people have become less willing to invest time, money, and energy in family life, turning instead to investments in themselves" (Popenoe, 1993, p. 527). This particular scholar has gone on to perpetuate the argument that the institution of family is in decline. To strengthen families, he suggests that we need to return to a traditional model of one partner being a wage earner and the other caring for the children and other dependent family members. What this model of family life does not adequately address is the concern that one family member will, thus, be economically vulnerable. Most households in the United States are either dependent on multiple incomes or are composed of only one head of household who needs to be in the paid labor force (McGraw & Walker, 2004). Embedded in the suggestion that we need to return to more "traditional" arrangements is the notion that women are at fault for the "decay" of society, as their appropriate role should be as primary caretakers of the home and family.

In the United States, opponents of a traditional distribution of roles in families advocate a family institution that is less hierarchically organized, that allows for greater personal growth for its members, and that encourages women to pursue educational and employment opportunities that benefit both individuals and society as a whole. From this perspective, public policy needs to be restructured to provide greater social benefits such as adequate child care, universal health insurance and flexible work schedules to accommodate caregiving and formal labor-force participation.

Much of this debate has ignored some other complicated issues that characterize contemporary times. For example, both advocates for "traditional" families and their critics have ignored the reality that increased educational opportunities and participation in the formal and informal labor force have allowed only certain groups of women to acquire the necessary economic resources to postpone marriage, to gain greater power vis-à-vis their spouse in marriage, and to leave abusive and exploitive marriages. For many other women, particularly those at the lower end of the socioeconomic scale, participating in the formal and informal labor force has not led to self-empowerment and autonomy. Instead, their employment outside of the home or away from traditional means of subsistence has translated into low-paying and, at times, risky jobs with schedules that interfere with child rearing. At times, their economic engagement has come at a high personal cost. Men socialized into "traditional" social roles may become embittered and downright abusive due to feelings of inadequacy about not fulfilling their provider role. This leads to violence toward women and their children in families and is an often overlooked phenomenon.

The "family values" debates combined with statistics on the high number of women in the paid labor force has spurred strident debates around parenting issues, social policies to support working parents, optimal conditions for child development, and socialization into "appropriate" gender roles. However, the cultural, political, and economic contexts within which these debates are held differ widely and elicit at times very diverse responses. It is thus impossible to speak just of one type of family experience as normative for all children.

THE SOCIALIZATION OF CHILDREN IN FAMILIES

Families are the primary vehicles of socialization for children, and virtually every aspect of their future lives is affected by these initial experiences (Karoly, Kilburn, & Cannon, 2005). Socialization involves learning the roles, norms, and values of a certain culture and society. Extensive research indicates that very early experiences are formative for individual development. Infants attain their first sense of self, other people, and social relationships through their initial interactions with their primary caregivers. While in the United States, we have emphasized the role of the mother in early socialization and development, there is an increasing scholarly and popular realization that fathers, siblings, and other closely involved individuals also provide crucial role models as well as nurturance for young children (Palkovitz, 2002).

An extensive literature around the socialization of children in families has centered on parenting styles, children's psychological makeup, intensive mothering, and father involvement. But perhaps none has been more controversial in recent years in the United States than the issue of gender socialization. Gender socialization refers to the process, assumed to start at birth, whereby cultural roles are learned according to one's sex. Cross-cultural evidence indicates that at times, even pre-birth, the fetus is treated differently if it is a boy or a girl (McHale, Crouter, & Tucker, 2003). Research indicates that depending on its sex, parents, caregivers, siblings, and other community members react to the young infant child differently, teaching it from birth that there are gender differences and that this behavior is accompanied by differing societal expectations for girls and boys. Children are directed into specific gender roles that impact their daily activities, the course of their lives, and their future potential. Extensive research indicates that despite dramatic changes, socialization differentiated by gender remains intact and, in fact, increases as young people enter adolescence (McHale, Crouter, & Tucker, 2003).

As children transition from childhood into adolescence, parents continue to play a significant role with respect to socialization. However, during this period, most teens also tend to seek out others, and peer influence grows in importance. While recent years have witnessed much debate about the significance of peers on adolescents, recent work indicates that effective parenting is directly related to decreased negative influence of peers and delinquency among adolescents (Simons, Chao, Conger, & Elder, 2001). Furstenberg (2000) has pointed out that much of the work on adolescents has approached this period of time in individuals' lives from a problem perspective, concentrating on deviant behavior creating the impression that all teens are plagued by problem behaviors. He points out that this is not necessarily the case, and that we need to look at the teenage years also as a period of positive development and growth. During this time in their lives, adolescents increasingly spend more time with peers, in school, and community settings, and are thus influenced by new ideas and perspectives. Today, more than ever before, teens are also inundated by media messages and communication technologies that facilitate networking across cultural and geographic boundaries. This connectivity translates into parental and familial socialization influences being in direct competition with other messages from external sources. However, there is much variation among adolescents with respect to personality and receptivity to multiple stimuli. It thus behooves us not to generalize and assume that all teens are vulnerable to negative messages or that family influence necessarily diminishes during this period. As with all other parts of the life course, a great deal of individual differences and situational experiences play a critical part in development.

Another significant aspect of socialization and an issue of major concern to many researchers and policy makers is the number of children being raised in single-parent homes. As of 2009, approximately 40 percent of children in the United States were born to unmarried mothers. *The 2009 Statistical Abstract of the United States* illustrates that about 30 percent, or 22 million, children under the age of 18 were not living with both parents last year. Most of these children lived with their mothers, while 3.5 percent lived not with either parent, but instead most probably with other relatives. Statistics also indicate that while most white children are born into two-parent households, divorce or an absent parent leads to about 21 percent of children not living with both parents. In comparison, 62 percent of black children were born to single mothers. About 30 percent of Hispanic children lived with only one parent; some of these parents were divorced, some were never married, and some had an absent father. These statistics indicate that for children born in the 1990s and 2000s, the likelihood is high that they will experience one-parent families at some point in their lives before they turn 18. One-parent families differ significantly from two-parent families due to changes in parenting styles and an increase in domestic and caretaking responsibilities for children (Jayakody & Kalil, 2002). Moreover, economics often play an important detrimental role in single-parent families as there is usually less money available to the mother and her children after the divorce.

In particular, single parenthood combined with poverty affects the lives of too many American children, and this is particularly true for children with disabilities. Approximately 29 percent of families headed specifically by single mothers live below the poverty line, compared to 8 percent of children living in two-parent families (Amato & Maynard, 2007), making their children more vulnerable to a wide array of risk factors (DeNavas-Walt, Proctor, & Smith, 2009). Analysis of longitudinal data indicates that approximately 34 percent of American children will spend at least one year of their lives living under the poverty level (Rank & Hirschi, 1999). It is important to note that, as multiple studies indicate, it is not necessarily single parenthood that is detrimental for children's development, but instead it is the combination of factors such as single parenthood combined with poverty, bad neighborhoods, and poor schools that influence child outcomes (Repetti, Taylor, & Seeman, 2002).

CHILDREN AND THE CHILD CARE CONTROVERSY

As the number of dual-earner families grows and single parenthood becomes more prevalent, child care arrangements have become one of the primary concerns for many American families. Approximately 76 percent of children under the age of 5 with working parents participate in some type of nonparental care, and two out of five have multiple care arrangements. Thus, parents and children negotiate a complex web of child care arrangements that include babysitters, child care centers, relatives, and friends. Moreover, about 41 percent of these children are in nonparental care at least 35 hours per week. A third of these children are put into non-arental care by the time they are 3 months old (Capizzano & Adams, 2000). These statistics, combined with the high percentage of women in the labor force, have fueled an intense debate in the United States about the role of families, specifically mothers, in children's lives, the effects of child care on children's development, and the role that the government should play with respect to the public financing of child care programs.

Complicating this debate is that studies on the effects of child care on children have proven that it is not necessarily the mother's working or nonparental child care that is problematic, but instead the quality of the programming that children are exposed to that matters most. For example, one national study found that only 10 percent of child care facilities for very young children could be rated as "excellent" (U.S. Consumer Product Safety Commission, 2001). These types of findings continue to raise parental concerns about the safety and the effects of nonparental care on children. In contrast, other studies have illustrated that when children from low-income families are placed in high-quality child care, they tend to outperform all children who have not been exposed to this type of learning situation by the time they enter kindergarten (NICHD, 2000). For example, high-quality child care in the first three years of a child's life leads to significant improvements in language ability and school readiness (NICHD, 2003). Early intervention programs such as Head Start also have been proven effective in mitigating some of the detrimental influences that young children in poverty experience. Children who have participated in high-quality child care are less likely to drop out of school once they are older and exhibit stronger language and mathematical skills than their counterparts who have attended programs of lesser quality (Reynolds, Temple, Robertson, & Mann, 2001). Extensive research continues on this question.

Those child care facilities that are associated with the strongest positive results for child outcomes tend to be small in size and to have a high adult-to-child ratio. However, two significant issues influence the provision of quality child care: (1) good child care is extremely expensive, making it inaccessible to the majority of American families; and (2), child care providers are among the poorest-paid professionals in U.S. society, often earning minimum wage with no retirement and health care benefits, though with the passage of health reform in 2010, these workers were intended to have health insurance by 2014. The impact on acquiring health insurance on the cost of child care is currently not known; however, it is believed that costs will increase in many instances and decrease in others. This leads to high turnover in child care facilities (by some estimates about 30 percent leave every year), affecting the quality of programming that is delivered to children (Zuckerman, 2000). These various issues make affordable, quality child care one of the primary problems facing contemporary American families.

CHILDREN AND DIVORCE

It has now become commonplace for children in the United States to experience the divorce of their parents and to live apart usually from their father. Approximately 40 percent of children under the age of 18 will experience the divorce of their parents, and another subset will experience a remarriage and subsequent divorce. Many of these families are or become economically vulnerable, and they are represented disproportionally by ethnic and racial minorities. Many studies have found that while not necessarily permanently damaging, divorce does have a significant impact on children's academic success and social development (Amato, 2002). What is often not clearly explained through demographic studies of divorce is that it is the actual long-term divorce process that can prove to be so detrimental for children. Divorce is usually the culmination of a whole series of family problems rather than just the starting point. Research indicates that boys in particular tend to suffer from familial conflict long before the actual divorce occurs. Moreover, many couples that ultimately separate engage in a series of detrimental behaviors before the divorce, such as poor parenting practices and high levels of conflict. They are often less involved in their children's educational and social lives, leading to behavior problems in their offspring (Furstenberg, 2009).

Problem behaviors in children are often compounded after a divorce primarily because of poor parenting practices, financial issues, and multiple transitions. A primary factor that influences children's negative behaviors is that many parents do not supervise their children properly once they leave their marriage, engage in poor parent-child relationships, and expose their children to open conflicts with their ex-spouse. Research has shown that when parents make a conscious effort, they can minimize the effects of divorce on their children by keeping both parents engaged with the children, offering guidance and advice, and limiting their exposure to conflict and negativity about the nonresidential parent (Amato, 2002). Finances also seriously affect the divorce process. Mothers are often hardest hit, as their income drops by about a third after a divorce due to women's lesser earnings and often a lack of child support. Financial and emotional strains compound after a divorce, taking a toll particularly on the parent with whom the child or children live and their children. Many women and their children also move from their residential home, causing a disruption of social support networks. Research indicates that responses to divorce differ by gender, with boys acting out through arguments and anger, and girls becoming more depressed and anxious (Morrison & Cherlin, 1995). Over time, many children also lose contact with their nonresidential parent, usually the father.

Over the long term, most children recover from the negative repercussions of divorce. While Judith Wallerstein's work (Wallerstein, Lewis, & Blakeslee, 2000) has received much media press for its findings that divorce irreparably harms a significant number of children as they move into adulthood, many other studies have disproven her thesis and have suggested instead that it is the coming together of factors such as poverty and parental negativity that can harm children over the long term. For example, Hetherington and Kelly (2002) report from their investigations that approximately 80 percent of children of divorce eventually adapt to the situation and proceed to have successful lives. This is not to suggest that divorce is not immensely difficult for all those involved, but only to point out that most individuals are able to cope with the changed familial circumstances and to move on in life. The research on the resilience of children is encouraging. Moreover, a small subset of studies has found that the consequences for children experiencing continued conflict between their parents is actually more detrimental to their long-term development than had their parents divorced (Amato & Booth, 1997).

Children who seem to fare best after a divorce are those who have been exposed to a minimum of conflict pre- and post-divorce and who receive a great deal of social support from their families and friends. Custodial and noncustodial parents need to provide emotional responsiveness, show involvement in the children's activities, and keep their children out of their battles (Leon, 2003).

Interestingly, research indicates that there is no real benefit for children when parents remarry. While remarriage introduces a new parental figure into the household and may enhance financial well-being, children in remarried families exhibit the same degree of behavioral problems as children in single-parent families and often deal with more interpersonal conflicts than children being raised in their original two-parent families (Garnefski & Diekstra, 1997).

CONCLUDING THOUGHTS AND POLICY IMPLICATIONS

Empirical evidence indicates that families continue to function as a source of resilience for children, and that the extent to which families mitigate risk factors plays a crucial role in children's developmental outcomes. Despite some claims that environmental and peer influences are stronger influences on children's development, research indicates that parents provide material and social capital for their children, act as buffers between their children and harmful environmental influences, and continue throughout a child's life course to influence its emotional, physical, and social well-being. This crucial relationship is basic to understanding any aspect of a child's life and needs to be considered in analyses that attempt to posit that race, ethnicity, socioeconomic status, religion, and disabilities are equal or more important variables.

Clarke-Stewart (2006) identifies the following factors as basic to rethinking policies that would further children's development: (1) it is not necessarily just poverty that is a risk factor for children, but instead it is the *number* of risks that a child is exposed to that is detrimental; (2) fathers matter as much as mothers with respect to child outcomes;

(3) family dynamics are closely correlated with child outcomes no matter how much time a child spends in child care; (4) divorce combined with poor parenting can have long-term detrimental effects on children; and (5) consistent conflict in families has negative repercussions for children. She goes on to explain that research findings such as these need to be viewed through a policy lens that promotes protective qualities in children themselves (such as academic achievement, strong attachments to caregivers, and positive relationship skills) and that give children the chance to find support and success in a range of settings and experiences (such as home, school, community, and peers). This strengths-based perspective advocates that instead of intervening only once problems have set in, we need to develop and encourage new perspectives and policies that have broad holistic impacts and that implement a preventative approach. Instead of targeting specific groups of children, or just schools or families, policies need to be put in place that support and encourage the competencies of all children. Moreover, if limited resources are at issue, the scholarly literature on risk and resilience suggests that policies that target young children at risk tend to be more effective than intervening later on in life (Clarke-Stewart, 2006).

We also need to be aware of the fact that different families are going to have varying needs and be exposed to a range of risk factors. This makes it difficult to speak of one specific family policy or set of policies. However, we can identify social or life domains that need to be reorganized in such a manner that they will enhance the quality of life for families and their children. For example, work needs to be restructured to allow parents to have more control over their time, to allow for job sharing, and/or to work from home. In addition, since child care has become such a crucial part of most American families' lives, it would be immensely beneficial if government were to regulate and support quality child care. Current regulatory policy and practice is divided between state and federal governments, and there is enormous variation among and between the states. Children who grow up in high-risk areas are now known to profit from an array of social services with respect to health care and education. Thus, we need to subsidize and build up these structures so that they can assist families with their quest to raise children with positive developmental outcomes.

What the scholarship on children and families ultimately tells us is that while family forms and risk factors differ, as long as children have loving, involved caregivers, they flourish. In the final analysis, the single most important factor that can optimize child outcomes is the quality of the parent-child relationship. Thus, we need to aim our policies toward promoting supportive environments that give parents the tools to promote the positive well-being of their children. This requires supporting families from an economic and social perspective, especially those who are most vulnerable and who have severe financial needs. Investing in children and their families right from the start is actually more cost-effective than attempting to intervene further on down the road when severe problems have set in. In sum, supporting families allows us to create more optimal environments for children and to mitigate so many of the factors that can ultimately undermine the healthy development of young people in our society.

REFERENCES

Amato, P. (2002). The consequences of divorce for adults and children. In R. Milardo (Ed.), *Understanding families into the new millennium: A decade in review* (pp. 488–506). Minneapolis: National Council on Family Relations.

Amato, P., & Booth, A. (1997). *A generation at risk: Growing up in an ear of family upheaval*. Cambridge, MA: Harvard University Press.

Amato, P., & Maynard, R. (2007, Fall). Decreasing nonmarital births and strengthening marriage to reduce poverty. *The Future of Children, 17*(2).

Bengston, V. L., & Allen, K. R. (1993). The life course perspective applied to families over time. In P. Boss, W. Doherty, R. LaRossa, W. Schumm, & S. Steinmetz (Eds.), *Sourcebook of family theories and methods: A contextual approach* (pp. 469–499). New York: Plenum.

Bianchi, S., Robinson, J., & Milkie, M. (2007). *Changing rhythms of American family life*. New York: Russell Sage Foundation.

Bromley, J., Hare, D., Davison, K., & Emerson, E. (2004). Mothers supporting children with autistic spectrum disorders: Social support, mental health status, and satisfaction with services. *Autism, 8*, 409–423.

Buck, F., Van Wel, F., Knijn, T., & Hagendoorn, L. (2008). Intergenerational contact and the life course status of young adult children. *Journal of Marriage and Family, 70*, 144–156.

Capizzano, J., & Adams, G. (2000). The number of child care arrangements used by children under five: Variation across states. Urban Institute. http://www.newfederalism.urban.org/pdf/anf_b12pdf

Cherlin, A. (2010). *Public and private families: An introduction*. New York: McGraw Hill.

Clarke-Stewart, A. (2006). What have we learned: Proof that families matter, policies for families and children, prospects for future research. In A. Clarke-Stewart & J. Dunn (Eds.), *Families count: Effects on child and adolescent development* (pp. 321–336). New York: Cambridge University Press.

Coontz, S. (1992). *The way we never were: American families and the nostalgia trap*. New York: Basic Books.

DeNavas-Walt, C., Proctor, B., & Smith, J. (2009). Income, poverty, and health insurance coverage in the United States: 2008. In *Current Population Reports, P60-236 (RV)*. Washington, DC: U.S. Government Printing Office.

Fischer, C., & Hout, M. (2010). The family in trouble: Since when? For whom? In. A. Cherlin (Ed.), *Public and Private Families*. New York: McGraw Hill.

Furstenberg, F. (2000). The sociology of adolescence and youth in the 1990s: A critical commentary. *Journal of Marriage and the Family, 62*, 896–910.

Furstenberg, F. (2009). If Moynihan had only known: Race, class and family change in the late twentieth century. *Annals of the American Academy of Political and Social Science, 631*, 94–110.

Garnefski, N., & Diekstra, R. (1997). Adolescents from one parent, stepparent, and intact families: Emotional problems and suicide attempts. *Journal of Adolescence 20*, 201–208.

Gates, G., Badgett, J., Macomber, J., & Chambers, K. (2007, March). *Adoption and foster care by gay and lesbian parents in the United States*. Urban Institute. Retrieved January 20, 2010, from http://www.urban.org

Hartmann, H. (1981). The family as the locus of gender, class and political struggle: The example of housework. *Signs, 6*, 366–394.

Hattery, A. (2001). *Women, work and family: Balancing and weaving*. London: Sage.

Hetherington, E., & Kelly, J. (2002). *For better or for worse: Divorce reconsidered*. New York: W. W. Norton.

Jayakody, R., & Kalil, A. (2002). Social fathering in low-income African American families with preschool children. *Journal of Marriage and Family, 64*, 504–516.

Joesch, J. M., & Smith, K. R. (1997). Children's health and their mothers' risk of divorce or separation. *Social Biology, 44*(3–4), 159–169.

Karoly, L. A., Kilburn, M. R., & Cannon, J. S. (2005). *Early childhood interventions: Proven results, future promise*. Santa Monica, CA: RAND Corporation.

Leon, K. (2003). Risk and protective factors in young children's adjustment to parental divorce: A review of the research. *Family Relations, 52*, 258–270.

Masnick, B., & Bane, M. J. (1980). *The Nation's Families 1960–1990*. Boston: Auburn House.

McGraw, L., & Walker, A. (2004). Gendered family relations: The more things change, the more they stay the same. In M. Coleman & L. Ganong (Eds.), *Handbook of contemporary families: Considering the past, contemplating the future* (pp. 174–191). Thousand Oaks, CA: Sage Publications.

McHale, S., Crouter, C., & Tucker, C. (2003). Family context and gender role socialization in middle childhood: Comparing girls to boys and sisters to brothers. *Child Development 70*(4), 990–1004.

Moen, P., & Sweet, S. (2003). Time clocks: Work-hour strategies. In P. Moen (Ed.), *It's about time: Couples and careers*. Ithaca, NY: Cornell University Press.

Morrison, D., & Cherlin, A. (1995). The divorce process and young children's well-being: A prospective analysis. *Journal of Marriage and the Family, 57*, 800–812.

NICHD Early Child Care Research Network. (2000). Characteristics and quality of child care for toddlers and preschoolers. *Journal of Applied Developmental Science, 4*, 116–135.

NICHD Early Child Care Research Network. (2003). Does amount of time in child care predict socioemotional adjustment? *Child Development, 74*, 976–1005.

Palkovitz, R. J. (2002). *Involved fathering and men's adult development: Provisional balances*. Hillsdale, NJ: Lawrence Erlbaum Press.

Parish, S., Rose, R., Andrews, M., Grinstein-Weiss, M., Richman, E., & Dababnah, S. (2009) Material Hardship in US Families Raising Children with Disabilities: Research Summary & Policy Implications, *Research Brief*, University of North Carolina School of Social Work, 1–8.

Popenoe, D. (1993). American family decline, 1960–1990: A review and appraisal. *Journal of Marriage and the Family, 55*, 527–555.

Rank, M., & Hirschi, T. (1999). The economic risk of childhood in America: Estimating the probability of poverty across the formative years. *Journal of Marriage and the Family, 61*, 1058–1067.

Repetti, R. L., Taylor, S. E., & Seeman, T. E. (2002). Risky families: Family social environments and the mental and physical health of offspring. *Psychological Bulletin, 128*, 330–366.

Reynolds, A., Temple, J., Robertson, D., & Mann, E. (2001). Long-term effects of an early childhood intervention on educational achievement and juvenile arrest: A 15-year follow-up of low-income children in public schools. *Journal of the American Medical Association, 285*, 2339–2346.

Rupp, K., & Ressler, S. (2009) Family caregiving and employment among parents of children with disabilities on SSI. *Journal of Vocational Rehabilitation, 30*, 153–175.

Saad, L. (2006, May). Americans have complex relationship with marriage. *Gallup monthly poll*. http://www.gallup.com/poll/23041/Americans-Complex-Relationship-Marriage.aspx

Seward, E. (1978). *The American family: A demographic history*. Beverly Hills, CA: Sage Publications.

Simons, R., Chao, W., Conger, R., & Elder, G. (2001). Quality of parenting as mediator of the effect of childhood deviance on adolescent friendship choices and delinquency: A growth curve analysis. *Journal of Marriage and Family, 63*, 63–79.

Smith, D. E. (1993). The standard North American family: SNAF as an ideological code. *Journal of Family Issues, 14*, 50–65.

Stacey, J. (1996). *In the name of the family: Rethinking family values in the post-modern age*. Boston: Beacon Press.

U.S. Census Bureau. (2008). Table 58: Households, families, subfamilies, and married couples. In *The 2008 statistical abstract*, http://www.2010census.biz/compendia/statab/cats/population/households_families_group_quarters.html

U.S. Census Bureau. (2009). Table 68: Children under 18 years old by presence of parents. In *The 2009 statistical abstract*. http://www.2010census.biz/compendia/statab/cats/population/households_families_group_quarters.html

U.S. Consumer Product Safety Commission. (2001). *Home playground equipment-related deaths and injuries*. Washington, DC: Author. http://www.cpsc.gov/library/playground.pdf

U.S. Department of Labor. (2009). *Women in the labor force: A databook*, Report 1018. http://www.bls.gov/cps/wlf-databook2009.htm

Wallerstein, J., Lewis, J., & Blakeslee, S. (2000). *The unexpected legacy of divorce*. New York: Hyperion.

Wymbs, B., Pelham, W., Molina, B., Gnagy, E., Wilson, T., & Greenhouse, J. (2008). Rate and predictors of divorce among parents of youths with ADHD. *Journal of Consulting and Clinical Psychology, 76,* 435–744.

Yamada, A., Suzuki, M., Kato, M., Suzuki, M., Tanaka, S., Shindo, T., et al. (2007). Emotional distress and its correlates among parents of children with pervasive developmental disorders. *Psychiatry and Clinical Neurosciences, 61,* 651–657.

Zuckerman, D. (2000). *Child care staff: The low-down on salaries and stability.* National Center for Policy Research for Women & Families. http://www.center4policy.org/wwf2.html

Chapter 7

Program Evaluation in Early Intervention and Early Childhood Special Education

Susan P. Maude and Lizanne DeStefano

Program evaluation is the process of carefully collecting information about a program or some aspect of a program to guide improvement, judge its quality or impact, or make management decisions (McNamara, 2010; Raizen & Rossi, 1981; Wholey, Hatry, & Newcomer, 1994; Weiss, 1997). In this chapter, we will refer to early childhood programs including, but not limited to, those funded by public schools, public state agencies (Departments of Education, Health and Human Services), private and/or not-for-profit, corporate funding operations, and community organizations. Furthermore, this chapter will focus on the assessment of *programs* not on individual child or family assessment.

Program evaluation includes a wide array of approaches, such as needs assessments, accreditation, cost-benefit analysis, effectiveness, formative (during the operation of a program), summative (at the end of a program), goal-based, process, outcomes, impact, and so on (Chen, 2005; Donaldson, Christie, & Mark, 2009; Killion, 2007; Stake, 2003; Worthen & Sanders, 1987). The type of evaluation approach one chooses depends on what one wants to learn about a program and the use to which evaluation information will be put. In the past decade, evaluation efforts in early intervention and early childhood special education (EI/ECSE) have focused heavily on accountability and accreditation. One reason for the emphasis on accountability was the priority placed on outcomes data by the Office of Management and Budget (OMB), one of the largest agencies within the Executive Office, as well as the

Government Performance and Results Act (GPRA) of 1993 (Harbin, Rous, & McLean, 2005). These federal initiatives were one of the first to require all federal programs to report "data on progress toward meeting the goals of the program, which in turn are used to help determine federal budget allocations" (Rous, McCormick, Gooden, & Townley, 2007, p. 20). In this chapter, we move beyond that focus and encourage additional uses for program evaluation and building the capacity of and climate for evaluation in EI/ECSE programs.

Many practical factors shape the evaluation, including the consumer or client (family, funder, board of directors) need for information, timeline for use of results, resources available, access to evaluation expertise, audience and stakeholder expectations, data collection, and analysis capacity. Before beginning an evaluation, these factors should be thoroughly explored by the client in collaboration with key stakeholders including program staff, and considered in every aspect of evaluation planning. For example, if evaluation information is needed in six months to serve as the basis for an application for refunding, then the design of the evaluation must ensure that the evaluation will produce findings for use by that date. Elaborate designs that will take longer than six months to produce results, though attractive, are not appropriate for this purpose. Likewise, if local capacity to collect and report data is limited, evaluation planning must take that into consideration by either building in data collection training and support into the design, bringing in external expertise, or employing data collection methods that are aligned with local capacity.

This chapter will argue for the need for a conceptual framework to help guide an evaluation, provide a brief overview of five evaluation frameworks that have strong applicability to early childhood programs, discuss issues in planning and conducting evaluation of EI/ECSE programs, and provide information about participatory designs. Our purpose is to encourage EI/ECSE programs to expand upon accountability efforts currently mandated by state or federal funding agencies to collect information on program effectiveness and program quality that is more useful for program improvement and impact assessment. As reported by Meisels (2007), evaluation in early childhood must move beyond mere outcome assessment for accountability purposes to a fuller analysis of the effectiveness of program elements, pedagogy, curriculum, and child outcomes to determine what works for whom and to guide program improvement.

USE OF A CONCEPTUAL FRAMEWORK TO DRIVE AN EVALUATION

Whether you are evaluating local, regional, state, national, and/or international programs, a conceptual framework is essential to a coherent, transparent, rigorous evaluation. A conceptual framework can show relationships among the components of the EI/ECSE program (e.g., philosophical underpinnings, screening, assessment, curricula, staffing, family support, fee structure for peers with typical development) and the intended outcomes. As such, the conceptual framework guides the choices to be made at each step in an evaluation. Development of the framework forces the evaluation team to be explicit from the outset about their assumptions regarding what will be measured, why it is being measured, and how the data will be analyzed and reported. Therefore, this step ensures that, at the end of the process, findings will meet the intended information needs. Moreover, a conceptual framework provides a structure for understanding, interpreting, and manipulating outcome measures. It answers the question of why a particular outcome is important, and identifies factors that must be taken into account to be able to interpret results appropriately. The conceptual framework is critical to the success of an evaluation and should be specified in as much detail as possible (DeStefano & Wagner, 1992; Greene, Caracelli, & Graham, 1989; Stecher & Davis, 1987). Studies have been conducted reviewing evaluation of human services (Halpern, 1987) and found that despite the recommendation that they begin with the articulation of a conceptual model that describes the major elements of the program and guides the development of the evaluation design, many studies continue to fail to make explicit the conceptual frameworks underlying the program theory and operations.

Advantages for using a conceptual framework include the following: (1) it identifies advance organizers and any major questions the evaluation should address (individual and overall), thereby guiding the evaluation; (2) it provides a visual or graphic representation of process and product portions of your efforts and any possible causal connections; (3) it clarifies each element of your EI/ECSE program and/or efforts; (4) it helps insure that what is being evaluated is indeed what should be evaluated; and (5) it serves as a means to share with others the complexities of your work.

The lack of a conceptual framework can seriously limit the usefulness of the evaluation findings. Time and effort can be expended on the collection of data that may not relate to what the "stakeholders" are trying to measure or impact. A stakeholder is defined as any individual who may have a vested interest or "stake" in the program. Stakeholders in an EI/ECSE program could include but are not limited to administrators, staff, children, family members, funders, and community partners. Stakeholders or funders may experience frustration when the questions for which they need answers are not addressed.

The next section of this chapter will focus on five particular evaluation approaches or frameworks that assist EI/ECSE programs in making decisions about their program: (1) goal-based, (2) standards-based, (3) outcome-impact, (4) consumer-oriented or participatory, and (5) cost-benefit analysis.

Goal-Based Evaluation

Goal-based evaluations are a useful framework to implement when determining if an EI/ECSE program has met its predetermined goals or objectives (McNamara, 2010; Stecher & Davis, 1987). This approach to evaluation is also referred to as goal-oriented evaluation and has similarities to the outcomes-based evaluation to be reviewed later in this chapter. Often EI/ECSE programs are established to meet one or more specific goals. These goals are often described in the original program plans. Table 7.1 provides a good overview of questions to ask in developing your goal-based evaluation.

Methods

Goal-based evaluation can use a variety of methods to assess the extent to which the program is making progress toward attaining its

Table 7.1　An overview of questions to consider when developing a goal-based evaluation.

1. Implementation: Is the EI/ECSE program being implemented on schedule and as planned?
2. Effectiveness: Are key components of the EI/ECSE program operating effectively? How might they be improved?
3. Impact: What outcomes are associated with participation in the EI/ECSE program? How do these compare with a comparable group of children/families in other EC programs? What is the value-added of participation in the program?
4. Sustainability: How and to what extent are elements of the EI/ECSE program becoming a part of the regular operations and how will they be sustained? What opportunities and barriers exist?

stated goals, including surveys, interviews, direct assessments, observation, document review, and secondary analysis of existing data. The key to effective goal-based evaluation is that the program goals must be explicit, understood, and valued by key stakeholders. Goals must be measurable. If the goals are not stated in measurable terms or if there is no consensus around the goals, then goal-based evaluation is not a good choice to frame the evaluation.

Strengths and Limitations

Goal-based evaluation is a good choice for many EI/ECSE programs because it is straightforward and easily understood by those within and outside the program. It is an appropriate evaluation approach for programs at all stages of development. Formative information on progress toward stated goals is useful for program management and improvement, while summative information on program outcomes and impact can attest to program quality and effectiveness. As stated earlier, goal-based evaluation requires clear, agreed-upon, measurable goals. If these do not exist, goal-based evaluation should not be attempted until goals have been developed and adopted by an EI/ECSE program. A limitation to this type of program evaluation is that the focus of the evaluation is very narrow, specifically focused on the program goals, and other unintended goals may not be identified.

Exemplars in EI/ECSE

Prior to the emphasis on outcomes or standards, EI/ECSE programs were typically designed around particular goals (to support the EI/ECSE program in engaging parents as partners in their child's education) and subsequent activities to meet or obtain that goal (conduct a needs assessment survey, identify priorities from the results of the survey, and implement activities in support of those activities). The activities were then evaluated to determine how best they met the originally stated goals. Head Start and programs funded by not-for-profit agencies (The ARC) have typically utilized goal-based evaluations. Furthermore, professional development plans for educators and teachers may also embrace a goal-based evaluation approach.

Standards-Based Evaluation

Standards-based evaluation measures a program against a set of commonly accepted standards in the field. Pre-K Now (2009) defines standards as "a broad term referring to structural guidelines and requirements that form the basis of a pre-k system, all of which are important and inter-related" (para. 1). The structural guidelines and requirements from federal, state, and professional policy typically addresses the use of standards in EI/ECSE across three levels: (1) program, (2) professional, and (3) child or early learning.

The first level, program standards, includes the regulations that guide how EI/ECSE programs operate. The Division for Early Childhood (DEC) of the Council for Exceptional Children (CEC) is the leading professional organization for young children with diverse abilities and their families. In the 1980s, DEC identified recommended practices to guide service delivery in EI/ECSE. Little to no evidence exists that these practices are being used by practitioners in the field or have been embedded into higher education personnel preparation programs (Bruder & Dunst, 2005; Campbell, Chiarelo, Wilcox, & Milbourne, 2009; Dunst & Bruder, 2006). In 2003, the Early Childhood Outcomes (ECO) Center was funded by the U.S. Department of Education to assist states in developing high-quality EI/ECSE state systems (Early Childhood Outcomes Center, 2010). Accreditation or monitoring, sometimes referred to as continuous improvement, is a common evaluation approach in which a program is compared against a set of program standards.

The second level, professional standards, articulates the competencies and credentials needed by service providers and educators within the EI/ECSE programs. The Division for Early Childhood (DEC) of the Council for Exceptional Children (CEC) is the leading professional organization for young children with diverse abilities and their families. DEC has identified specific competencies or standards for educators who work in EI/ECSE settings at the initial or entry and advanced levels (DEC, 2008a,b). Institutes of higher education (IHEs) utilize these standards to design their professional development programs of study at the undergraduate and graduate levels. Furthermore, state departments of education have developed their state licensure and standards built upon these DEC competencies. Unfortunately, Bruder and her colleagues working from the Center to Inform Personnel Preparation, Policy, and Practice (2008) reported that IHEs and states responsible for licensure are inconsistent in their utilization of these competencies. Furthermore, she advocates for a national set of competencies in EI/ECSE (Bruder, 2010).

The third level, child or early learning standards, describe what children should know as a result of participating in an early childhood program (Pre-K Now, 2010).

Early learning standards are "widely accepted statements of expectations for children's learning" (Council of Chief State School Officers [CSSO], 2009). Scott-Little and her colleagues identified the content addressed by states in the development of infant-toddler early learning guidelines (Scott-Little, Kagan, Frelow, & Reid, 2009).

Standards-based evaluation differs from normative evaluation techniques because rather than comparing programs or schools to other programs or schools, they are measured against a standard of excellence. There are several types of standards. Content standards describe what a child should know or be able to do at a particular age or grade level in a particular content area. Curriculum standards specify what should be taught at a specific age or grade level rather than what students should know. Performance standards describe knowledge or skills that are assessed through the observation, description, or documentation of child behavior or performance in connection with broadly stated content standards. Standards are typically aligned to instruction, learning, and assessment in the classroom (CSSO, 2009; Kagan & Scott-Little, 2004).

Early learning standards are "statements that describe expectations for the learning and development of young children." These expectations may relate to several domains, such as physical well-being, social and emotional well-being, language development, approaches to learning, and general knowledge. These standards describe what knowledge, skills, and dispositions children at a certain age or developmental period are expected to know. They are designed to understand what knowledge teachers, programs, parents, and the community are expected to know so that they can help the children learn. Early learning standards are developed through researching early learning and development processes, sequences, and long-term consequences. They should be appropriate for and inclusive of the widest range of life situations and experiences possible (CSSO, 2009).

Methods

Standards-based evaluation generally comes with a set of prescribed methods to assess the extent to which the program is aligned with a particular set of standards. The key to effective standards-based evaluation is that the selected standards must be appropriate for achieving the intended goals of the program, aligned with program context, including populations served, and valued by key stakeholders and measurable.

Strengths and Limitations

Standards-based evaluation is a good choice for many EI/ECSE programs because it is straightforward, easily understood by those within and outside the program, and is appropriate for programs at all stages of development. Formative information on how a program embodies a common set of standards is useful for program management and improvement, while summative information on standards alignment is commonly accepted evidence of program quality and effectiveness. Programs may be confused by the proliferation of standards and have difficulty selecting those that are most appropriate for their evaluation needs.

Exemplar in EI/ECSE

Much effort has been expended by state departments of education to develop early learning standards for both the 0–3 age group of children with disabilities and the 3–5 age group of children with and without disabilities (Kagan & Scott-Little, 2004; Scott-Little et al., 2009). One particular state to highlight here has been Vermont. The Vermont Early Learning Standards, or VELS (2003), were developed by a subcommittee of the Vermont Early Childhood Work Group. Similar to work in other states, the standards were written using a four-tiered structure around (1) domains, (2) learning goals and definitions, (3) examples, and (4) supports for learning. Their strong commitment to the value and importance of play as a key component in the learning process is unique. Their statement about play and how they embedded its importance can be found on the first pages of the VELS document:

> **The Role of Play in Addressing the Standards:** The subcommittee acknowledged the important role of play in how children learn by including it as a guiding principle and as the first Learning Goal in each of the domains. There is abundant evidence that children learn best through play. The sub-committee based its thinking about each domain on the understanding that children should be provided with opportunities to play in a learning environment that addresses their developmental needs for movement, problem-solving, creativity, and social interaction with adults and other children. Teachers and families can best guide learning in all domains by providing opportunities for children to explore and apply new skills in natural contexts. Responsive adults teach young children by interacting through play with each child according to the child's interests, abilities, and

cultural preferences. Through play, children enhance the learning of skills, knowledge and dispositions that guarantees success in later schooling. In VELS, therefore, play is one way that children can achieve the Examples described in each of the eight learning Domains. (VELS, 2003, 2)

Outcome or Impact-Based Evaluation

Outcome evaluation is defined as the systematic collection of information to assess the impact of a program, present conclusions about the merit or worth of a program, and make recommendations about future program directions or improvements (CDC, 2007; Reisman, 1994; Reisman & Clegg, 2000; United Way of America, 1996; W. K. Kellogg Foundation [WKKF], 2004). Outcome-based evaluations are focused on determining, exploring, and describing changes that occur as a result of a program being implemented (Fitzpatrick, Sanders, & Worthen, 2004). An outcome is defined as a change in behavior, knowledge, understanding, ability, skill, or attitudes resulting from participation in a program or course, the receipt of services, or the use of a particular product (CSSO, 2009).

Outcome or impact evaluations may be either formative or summative and include consideration of outcomes that are immediate effects, expected final outcomes, and unintended outcomes (Fitzpatrick, Sanders, & Worthen, 2004; Hatry & Kopczynski, 1997; Westmoreland, Lopez, & Rosenberg, 2009). For example, formative outcome evaluations may determine what changes should be made to EI services or ECSE curricula to achieve desired outcomes, while summative evaluations determine whether goals are being sufficiently met to justify the continuation of funding to an innovative EI/ECSE program.

A preliminary step to a good evaluation is clearly articulating expected outcomes. As shown in Figure 7.1, a logic model is a useful

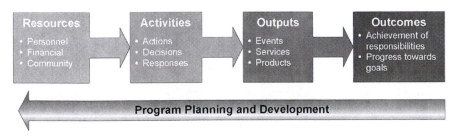

Figure 7.1 Logic model components.

mechanism for designing an evaluation based on an impact hypothesis. It is grounded in the assumption that, for an impact to be achieved, there are enabling conditions in the form of resources, inputs, activities, and outputs (Corso & Maude, 2008).

The use of the logic model framework for outcome evaluation is well documented[1] and has been applied to assess government projects, private industry, and human service programs. This approach has also been applied to early childhood programs and advocated by national early childhood technical assistance systems (NECTAC, OSEP). As the logic model illustrates, some of the initiative's outcomes pertain to expected changes at the individual level (generally immediate outcomes). Other outcomes pertain to changes at the community and workforce levels (generally termed intermediate outcomes).

The ability of program stakeholders to utilize the logic model throughout multiple stages of the program's "life" makes it even more valuable. The logic model may be used in program design, program implementation, and program evaluation. In program design, the model may be used to develop a program strategy and illuminate program concepts and goals for stakeholders, and guide the examination of research that may contribute to program development. In program implementation, the logic model provides focus on desired results and helps to identify information needs for program monitoring and enhancement for achieving these results. Finally, in program evaluation, the logic model provides a guide to the evaluative information needed to assess program impacts. Table 7.2 provides the basic terminology used in outcome evaluation, including the following: inputs/ resources, activities, outputs, outcomes, outcome indicator, outcome targets, and benchmarks.

Methods

The logic model framework is used to develop an understanding of the relationship between program resources, activities, and expected

---

[1]There are well over 100 references to logic model design and use in assessment in the literature. The Kellogg Foundation published and recently updated a comprehensive logic model development handbook, "Logic Model Development Guide: Logic models to bring together planning, evaluation & action" (2004). In addition, multiple government and research agencies, including the Centers for Disease Control, RAND, and United Way, have published evaluations and guidelines based on logic model theory.

Table 7.2   Glossary of Selected Outcome Measurement Terms

- **Inputs** are resources a program uses to achieve program objectives. Examples are the early childhood staff (early childhood teachers, para-educators, service providers, director), volunteers (foster grandparents, high school or college students), facilities, equipment, curricula, and money. An early childhood program uses its *inputs* to support its *activities*.

- **Activities** are what a program does with its inputs—the services it provides—to fulfill its mission. Examples are facilitating a half-day, four-day-a-week early childhood program, home visits, screening and assessment services, family education nights, adult education services, and/or providing adult mentors for youth. Program *activities* result in *outputs*.

- **Outputs** are products of a program's activities, such as the number of class sessions provided, number of adult education classes taught, number of children screened, or number of children/families served. Another term for "outputs" is "units of service." A program's *outputs* should produce desired *outcomes* for the program's participants.

- **Outcomes** are benefits for participants during or after their involvement with a program. Outcomes may relate to knowledge, skills, attitudes, values, behavior, condition, or status. Examples of outcomes include greater knowledge of nutritional needs, improved reading skills, more effective responses to conflict, getting a job, and having greater financial stability.

For a particular program, there can be various "levels" of outcomes, with initial outcomes or proximal outcomes leading to longer-term or distal ones. For example, a youth in a mentoring program who receives one-to-one encouragement to improve academic performance may attend school more regularly, which can lead to getting better grades, which can lead to graduating.

- **Outcome Indicators** are the specific items of information that track a program's success on outcomes. Many states have already identified key outcomes for communities to address by the time the child begins school at age 5. For instance, in Iowa there is a statewide "result" that children are ready to succeed in school. Two indicators of this "result" are (1) preliteracy skills, and (2) children in quality preschools.

They describe observable, measurable characteristics or changes that represent achievement of an outcome. For example, a program whose desired outcome is that participants pursue a healthy lifestyle could define "healthy lifestyle" as not smoking; maintaining a recommended weight, blood pressure, and cholesterol level; getting at least two hours of exercise each week; and wearing seat belts consistently. The number and percentage of program participants who demonstrate these behaviors, then, is an *indicator* of how well the program is doing with respect to the outcome.

- **Outcome Targets** are numerical objectives for a program's level of achievement on its outcomes. After a program has had experience with measuring outcomes, it can use its findings to set targets for the number and percentage of participants expected to achieve desired outcomes in the next

(Continued)

Table 7.2   (Continued)

reporting period. It also can set targets for the amount of change it expects participants to experience.

• **Benchmarks** are performance data that are used for comparative purposes. A program can use its own data as a baseline benchmark against which to compare future performance. It also can use data from another program as a benchmark. In the latter case, the other program often is chosen because it is exemplary and its data are used as a target to strive for, rather than as a baseline (United Way, 1996).*

*This list was modified from the United Way of America Model (1996) for an EI/ECSE setting.

outcomes using a systematic, visual representation (Kaplan & Garrett, 2005; WKKF, 2004). It provides stakeholders with a clearer understanding of how investments, both human and financial, may contribute to achieving program goals. There are five components to the basic logic model:

1. Resources, which include human, financial, organizational, and community inputs directed towards program use. In EI/ECSE settings, this could include early childhood personnel (years of experience, levels of education, types of education licenses or certifications, number of years in current position, ongoing professional development plans).
2. Program activities, which relate to how these inputs are used. This includes processes, events, actions, tools, and technology associated with implementation of the EI/ECSE program. Examples could include facilitating a half-day, four-day-a-week early childhood program, home visits, screening and assessment services, and family education nights.
3. Direct outputs, which may include multiple types and targets of service, are produced by the activities. Outputs are typically reported by numbers (number of home visits conducted, number of children screened and found eligible, number of families attending the family education nights). Previously, program evaluation efforts in EI/ECSE settings stopped at this level with the recording of outputs and numbers. However, the logic model proposes two additional components.
4. Outcomes, which identify specific changes in participant behavior, knowledge, status, skill, and level of functioning. Examples could include positive changes in child and/or adult behavior, knowledge, and skills as a result of the activities conducted and outputs achieved. These outcomes may be either

short term or long term, but generally occur within about seven years.

5. The final component of the basic logic model is program impact or the fundamental change occurring as a result of program activities. This impact may be either intended or unintended (references). An example of a program impact can be children prepared to enter kindergarten ready to learn.

Strengths and Limitations

Measurement of outcomes for evaluation is useful for four reasons:

1. Outcome evaluation allows EI/ECSE programs to track their own progress and identify possible weaknesses in need of improvement or additional focus.
2. EI/ECSE programs may use outcome information to develop budgets and justify spending.
3. Outcome information may also be used for public purposes in establishing educational accountability.
4. EI/ECSE programs may use the measurement of progress to communicate to families and the community the program's successes.

Benefits to conducting an outcome evaluation of an EI/ECSE program or services include the following: (1) strengthening of existing services; (2) targeting effective services for expansion; (3) identifying professional development needs; (4) developing and justifying budgets; and (5) preparing long-range plans. Limitations to using an outcome evaluation approach include the following: (1) findings of the outcome measurement does not reveal whether the outcomes being measured are the right ones; (2) without experimental or statistical controls, outcome measurements do not prove that the program caused the outcomes; (3) if an outcomes evaluation shows that participants are not experiencing benefits, it may not show where the problems lie; (4) some outcomes are difficult to measure, and (5) extra burden is placed on participants by having them complete surveys, participate in focus groups, etc.

Exemplar in EI/ECSE

This section will share two exemplars of a logic model. The first logic model is from a national parent involvement and education program entitled, Parents as Teachers (PAT). PAT is an early childhood parent education and family support system designed to empower families with the key outcome of helping all children to be healthy, safe, and ready to learn (PAT, 2010). PAT is a home visiting program and is replicated in nearly every state. The reader is guided to their Web site to review the logic model framework (http://www.parentsasteachers .org). The logic model graphic developed by PAT (found at http://www.parentsasteachers.org/images/stories/documents/LogicModel_2006.pdf) clearly guides the reader and stakeholders with a snapshot of the entire PAT program, beginning with key assumptions and values and ending with their intended outcomes.

The second logic model to showcase is currently utilized by a statewide ECSE professional development system in Illinois. Illinois STAR NET is a *S*upport and *T*echnical *A*ssistance *R*egional *NET*work that provides training, consultation, and resources to the early childhood community in Illinois. STAR NET has been in existence since the early 1990s, supported by funds from the U.S. Department of Education through the Illinois State Board of Education (Maude & Corso, in development). These professional development supports are targeted for families, educators, and related specialists who care for or provide services to young children with diverse abilities or disabilities. An additional graphic (see the first author, Susan Maude) captures the mission and activities of the STAR NET system as well as the immediate, intermediate, and long-term outcomes (Maude & Corso, 2010).

PAT and STAR NET provide very comprehensive yet different services with similar outcomes—better outcomes for young children and/or their families. The former program provides supports through home visitors who then work directly with families while the latter program offers ongoing professional development to families and other key early education and care providers to help children. These visuals serve as a means to clarify to others the very complicated yet value-added importance of these supports in the improvement of the lives of young children and their families.

Participatory/Consumer-Oriented Evaluation

The consumer-oriented approach assesses the extent to which a program meets the stated needs or concerns of consumers (children and families) rather than focusing on the extent to which a program meets its stated goals or aligns with a set of standards (Scriven, 1967; Vedung, 2000). In participatory evaluation, consumers and program staff are directly involved in planning and/or carrying out the evaluation as a means of ensuring that their needs are addressed and increasing their use of evaluation information. The consumer-oriented approach to evaluation is directed toward assessing educational programs, practices, and products with the informational needs of the consumer in mind (Fitzpatrick, Sanders, & Worthen, 2004; Scriven, 1973).

Methods

Consumer-oriented and participatory approaches generally involve collecting information directly from those served by the program using surveys, interviews, observations, and direct assessment of students, professionals, and families. A key aspect of data collection is to ensure that consumers are free to offer their perceptions of the program without consequence. This often involves the use of anonymous data collection procedures or third-party evaluators. In participatory evaluation, stakeholders may be involved in choosing methods, designing instruments, and collecting and reporting data.

Strengths and Limitations

One strength of the consumer-oriented approach is its unique focus on the consumer's information needs. Most evaluation approaches focus on the needs and expectations of those designing or administering the program, not those who consume the product being assessed (Fitzpatrick, Sanders, & Worthen, 2004). This approach is well aligned with the philosophy of family-centered practice and consumer involvement in EI/ECSE service provision. Consumer-oriented and participatory approaches also build capacity and empower consumers to take an active role in promoting quality services. Limitations of the consumer-oriented approach includes additional costs to the program and/or participants (time, money) in the development and implementation of the evaluation.

Exemplars in EI/ECSE

The Technical Assistance ALLIANCE for Parent Centers (the ALLIANCE) is an innovative partnership of one national and six regional parent technical assistance centers, each funded by the U.S. Department of Education's Office of Special Education Programs (OSEP). These seven projects comprise a unified technical assistance system for the purpose of developing, assisting, and coordinating the over 100 Parent Training and Information Centers (PTIs) and Community Parent Resource Centers (CPRCs) under the Individuals with Disabilities Education (IDEA) Act P.L. 108-446 (2004). The national and regional parent technical assistance centers work to strengthen the connections to the larger OSEP Technical Assistance and Dissemination Network and fortify partnerships between Parent Centers and education systems at local, state, and national levels (Alliance National Center, 2010).

Each state is home to at least one Parent Training and Information Center (PTIC). These centers serve families of children and young adults from birth to age 22 with all disabilities: physical, cognitive, emotional, and learning. "They help families obtain appropriate education and services for their children with disabilities; work to improve education results for all children; train and inform parents and professionals on a variety of topics; resolve problems between families and schools or other agencies; and connect children with disabilities to community resources that address their needs" (Alliance National Center, 2010).

The Alliance National Center uses a multi-level consumer oriented evaluation approach in which the six regional centers are surveyed and interviewed to determine the extent to which their needs are being met by the Alliance and randomly sampled state centers are interviewed to assess their level of interaction and satisfaction with the regional center. This consumer-oriented strategy is consistent with the needs-driven, service-oriented philosophy of the Parent Training Centers. National and regional centers used the evaluation results to improve consumer satisfaction and target services to meet expressed needs. Please see the Alliance Web site for more information (http://www.taalliance.org).

Cost-Benefit Analysis

Cost-benefit analysis involves identifying and determining the monetary value of the various costs and benefits associated with two or more well-defined alternatives (Fitzpatrick, Sanders, & Worthen, 2004; Goetze, 2007; Trefler, 2009). These costs and benefits are compared to determine which is greater, the costs or the benefits, and to what extent. This is then used to develop a benefit-to-cost ratio for each, the highest of which is then selected. A cost-benefit analysis may be conducted for two purposes (Gupta, 2001). First, one may assess whether the use of one program or activity yields greater benefit than an alternative program or activity. Second, one may also compare a particular project versus the option of making no changes or doing nothing (Gupta, 2001).

Since governments typically fund EI/ECSE programs (Barnett, 2000), it makes sense to evaluate the costs involved in operationalizing diverse early childhood delivery systems. A common argument in the field is that investment in early childhood development programs yield high levels of benefit to families and in state and federal spending. Early studies in the early childhood literature (Garland, Stone, Swanson, & Woodruff, 1981; Masse & Barnett, 2002; Schweinhart, Barnes, & Weikart, 1993) have documented positive benefits of early childhood programs, especially when programs that were of high quality, studies used a longitudinal design, and multiple effects were explored. It is interesting to note that in the last decade, more cost-benefit studies have emerged from researchers in the field of economics.

For example, a report published in 2003 reported an annual return of 16 percent for program participants and a 12 percent return for non-participants (Rolnick & Grunewald, 2003). These returns can be categorized into three groups: government budget benefits; increased earning and compensation; and decreased crime-associated cost for individuals. These returns vary in their level of immediacy. For example, decreased spending in special education is experienced sooner than decreased spending on crime, often found much later (Rolnick & Grunewald, 2003). It has also been found that programs directed at economically disadvantaged or impoverished families result in more immediate returns (Grunewald & Markeson, 2007; Lynch, 2007). These programs begin paying for themselves within six years in comparison to nine years for universal programs for 3- and 4-year-olds. This is because children from low-income environments are more likely to require special education and more likely to commit crimes (Grunewald & Markeson, 2007; Lynch, 2007).

Methods

Cost-benefit analyses are commonly done using six steps, as described by Gupta (2001). The first step, defining the goals of the project, is most easily done when the goals of the organization are clearly stated. This is because the evaluator can then more easily determine what action is required to achieve them. The second step is the identification of the alternatives to be evaluated. More difficult is determining what costs and benefits are associated with each alternative. The third step is to consider not only those costs and benefits that are both tangible and intangible, but also those that are direct and those that are indirect. Indirect costs and benefits affect the surrounding community or those outside of the participating group and often tend to be intangible.

The fourth and perhaps most difficult step in conducting a cost-benefit analysis is the estimation and valuation of costs and benefits. Accurately quantifying all costs and benefits related to the program is vital as it allows an evaluative conclusion to be reached once the assessment is completed. Unfortunately, many judgments and fallible estimates must be made.

The fifth and another difficult step relates to changes in these values over time. An assessor must determine whether each cost or benefit will change over time and, if so, to what extent. This requires a strong background in economics, such as an understanding of forecasted changes in supply and demand in specific markets in the future. Lastly, the sixth step builds upon information gathered in the past five steps, and requires the evaluator to determine which alternative yields the largest benefit to be ultimately recommended as the most favorable action to take (Gupta, 2001).

Strengths and Weakness

Having actual or "hard" data to support the financial commitment in support of EI/ECSE programs is a key strength for choosing a cost-benefit analysis. Knowing this information can assist policy makers when determining what level of funding is needed to obtain what types of impact (Barnett, 2000). Conducting a cost-benefit analysis poses certain challenges. There are many estimates of costs, benefits, and judgment calls to make, which often result in increased opportunity for error by the evaluator (Fitzpatrick, Sanders, & Worthen, 2004). Also, assessing the costs and benefits of a program often requires a strong knowledge of both the particular discipline of the program being evaluated and an understanding of technical issues and economic concepts. The assessor must understand the discipline to accurately identify all potential costs and benefits and to better understand how to convert these into monetary values. One must also understand the economic concepts to incorporate vital information such as current market conditions, economic trends in that time period or geographic area, and depreciation (Fitzpatrick, Sanders, & Worthen, 2004). Critical steps include asking the right questions and using the appropriate financial methods to yield accurate information (H. Meeks, personal communication, September 1, 2010).

Exemplars

Several states have conducted longitudinal cost-benefit analysis to determine what may be gained through increased investment in early childhood development programs. Between 1962 and 1989, over 100 families were tracked in a study conducted at the HighScope Perry Preschool Project in Ypsilanti, Michigan (Rolnick & Grunewald, 2003). The program paired daily 2½-hour classroom sessions with 1½-hour home visits and lasted 30 weeks annually. Teachers were well trained and paid 10 percent more than the standard pay for teachers in that school district. Furthermore, there was a 6:1 child-to-teacher ratio. At the age of 27, program participants were compared with a control group of nonparticipants, and significant results were found. Although cognitive advantages in the participating group leveled out within several years, participants were 20 percent more likely to complete high school, four times more likely to earn $2,000 or more monthly, and far less likely to be arrested five or more times.

A similar study was conducted at a Chicago Parent-Child (CPC) Center for families who are economically disadvantaged (Lynch, 2007; Reynolds, Temple, Robertson, & Mann, 2001). A study conducted between 1980 and 2004 investigated the long-term effects of program participation on participants with a comparable population of nonparticipants. Results showed that participants were less likely to be retained in a grade, require special education, be arrested, or experience abuse or neglect (Lynch, 2007). The author argues that these positive outcomes are in part a result of having well-trained teachers and a program emphasis on parental involvement. Ultimately, it was determined that the CPC program benefit-cost ratio is about 10–1. This means that every $1 spent on the program results in $10 of benefit. These benefits were calculated in the form of increased school performance and earning power and decreased crime and pain and suffering of crime victims.

Goetz and her colleagues at the Center for Persons with Disabilities in Utah have been evaluating the costs of both early intervention services (Part C) and most recently have begun investigating the impact of pre-K programs in New Mexico (2007). Having a background in economics certainly assists in this type of program evaluation.

OTHER ISSUES IN PLANNING AND CONDUCTING EVALUATIONS OF EARLY INTERVENTION AND EARLY CHILDHOOD SPECIAL EDUCATION PROGRAMS

In this chapter, we encourage those responsible for EI/ECSE programs to think beyond program evaluation for accountability purposes and to expand their program evaluation repertoire. Including conceptual frameworks and well-chosen evaluation approaches will provide more relevant information to guide program improvement or assess program quality, to communicate more effectively with stakeholders within and outside the program, and to build evaluation capacity among program staff, families, and other consumers. In these challenging economic times, EI/ECSE program administrators are likely to see evaluation as a necessary burden, rather than a way to engage program staff and build support for their program. However, when competition for funds is high, those programs with robust, useful evaluation strategies will be well positioned to argue for their effectiveness and well informed as to the best ways to restructure and respond to fiscal challenges.

Too often in early childhood programs and in education in general, we conduct evaluation because of external requirements and not because we see a real need or because we are truly interested in empirical answers to the questions, "How are we doing?" or "How can we improve?" A noble goal for an early childhood program is to embody the reflective practice that we try to instill in our teachers by embedding an effective and useful evaluation approach into the day-to-day functioning of the program. A routine question at staff meetings, planning sessions, and leadership retreats should be "What do we want to know about our program?" and to find ways to collect and review a variety of data (e.g., student progress, family involvement, consumer satisfaction, standards alignment) as a regular part of program management. Staff and administrators need support in developing their capacity to obtain data as well as learn how to utilize the data for continuous improvement efforts—not just to meet a funding requirement.

Program administrators who want to embed this kind of evaluation into their programs are quickly faced with challenges such as limited funding, lack of evaluation expertise, and time constraints. Creative solutions such as partnering with a university evaluation training program to involve graduate students in cost-effective evaluation projects, pooling evaluation resources with other EI/ECSE programs in your area to develop common instruments, databases, and other shared evaluation resources, and trading time and expertise by serving as "third-party" evaluators for other programs in exchange for their serving as evaluators for your program.

In programs that have a "culture of evaluation," program managers, board of directors, and staff engage regularly in evaluation as a vital part of program operations. Evaluation data are used routinely to guide planning and decision making. Key program stakeholders understand the theory or conceptual model that underlies the program and continually monitor the extent to which desired outcomes are attained. Building a "culture of evaluation" into early childhood programs takes considerable work, but can yield impressive benefits such as more effective, data-based decision making, continuous improvement resulting in enhanced outcomes and effectiveness, and greater collective understanding of and investment in high-quality programming for young children. Finally, existing resources are used more effectively in this framework.

It is important to acknowledge that some of the most important questions in early childhood programming cannot be answered by short-term, simplistic local evaluations. Seminal questions like, "Does this program make a difference in future educational outcomes for children in this community?" require longitudinal, development, multi-institutional collaborations, shared databases, and considerable analytic capacity. With the ESEA reauthorization, Race to the Top and State Fiscal Stabilization funding, and state and federal efforts to develop P-20 longitudinal data systems, we are beginning to develop an infrastructure within which these more ambitious and much-needed studies will become feasible in communities across the United States. Despite this promising development, it remains critical that early childhood professionals are actively involved in the creation and use of longitudinal data systems. Advocacy with local educational agencies, regional educational service centers, the state department of education, and state chapters of national professional associations is critical to ensuring that early childhood programs are represented accurately, that young child outcomes are well assessed, and that mechanisms for tracking children as they move from early intervention and preschool programs into K–12 and beyond yield desired results.

In summary, in recent years, the evaluation of early childhood education has been heavily dominated by accountability demands focused upon regulatory compliance and assessment of child outcomes, particularly academic and cognitive measures. In a time of greater competition for resources and increased demand for efficiency and effectiveness, new approaches to evaluation that promote high-quality programs, inform decision making, and demonstrate the impact and value-added of early childhood programming are essential. Partnerships with universities, K–12 schools, and professional associations can enhance local EI/ECSE programs capacity to enhance their evaluation capacity and adopt new approaches to formative and summative assessment. Advocacy at local, state, and federal levels is needed to ensure that early childhood programming is included in large-scale, longitudinal evaluation systems.

REFERENCES

Alliance National Center. (2010). Technical assistance ALLIANCE for parent centers national center (ALLIANCE). Retrieved from http://www.taalliance.org

Barnett, W. S. (2000). Economics of early childhood intervention. In J. P. Shonkoff & S. J. Meisels (Eds.), *Handbook of early childhood intervention* (2nd ed., pp. 589–610). New York: Cambridge University Press.

Bruder, M. B. (2010). Early childhood intervention: A promise to children and families for their future. *Exceptional Children, 76*(3), 339–355.

Bruder, M. B., & Dunst, C. J. (2005). Personnel preparation in recommended early intervention practices: Degree of emphasis across disciplines. *Topics in Early Childhood Special Education, 25*(1), 25–33.

Campbell, P. H., Chiarelo, L., Wilcox, M. J., & Milbourne, S. (2009). Preparing therapists as effective practitioners in early intervention. *Infants and Young Children, 22*(1), 21–31.

Center to Inform Personnel Preparation, Policy, and Practice (CIPPP). (2008). *Study VIII: Alignment of Early Childhood Special Education Higher Education Curriculum with National Personnel Standards and Certification Policies, 8*(1).

Centers for Disease Control (CDC). (2007). Evaluating outcomes of HIV prevention programs. Retrieved from http://www.cdc.gov/hiv/topics/evaluation/health_depts/guidance/outcome-eval.htm

Chen, H. T. (2005). *Practical program evaluation: Assessing and improving planning, implementation and effectiveness.* Newbury Park, CA: Sage Publications.

Corso, R. M., & Maude, S. P. (2008). NAEYC *Professional Development Division— Final Evaluation Repo*rt. Summative report developed for the National Association for the Education of Young Children (NAEYC).

Council of Chief State School Officers (CCSSO). (2009). *Early childhood glossary terms.* Retrieved from http://www.ccsso.org/Documents/2006/Assessing_Students_with_Disabilities_Glossary_2006.pdf

DeStefano, L., & Wagner, M. (1992). Outcome assessment in special education: What lessons have we learned? In F. Rusch, L. DeStefano, J. Chadsey-Rusch,

L. A. Phelps, & E. M. Szymanski (Eds.), *Transition from school to adult life: Models, linkages, and policy* (pp. 173–208). Sycamore, IL: Sycamore.

Division for Early Childhood (DEC). (2008a). *DEC ECSE-EI advanced ("Specialist") personnel standards w/ CEC advanced common core.* Missoula, MT: Author.

Division for Early Childhood (DEC). (2008b). *DEC ECSE-EI initial ("Professional") personnel standards w/ CEC common core.* Missoula, MT: Author.

Donaldson, S. I., Christie, C. A., & Mark, M. M. (2009). *What counts as credible evidence in applied research and evaluation practice?* Newbury Park, CA: Sage Publications.

Dunst, C. J., & Bruder, M. B. (2006). Early intervention service coordination models and service coordinator practices. *Journal of Early Intervention, 28*(3), 155–165.

Early Childhood Outcomes Center (ECO). (2010). *About ECO: Overview.* Retrieved from http://www.fpg.unc.edu/~eco/pages/overview.cfm

Fitzpatrick, J. L., Sanders, J., & Worthen, B. R. (2004). *Program evaluation: Alternative approaches and practical guidelines* (3rd ed.). Boston: Allyn & Bacon.

Garland, C., Stone, N. W., Swanson, J., & Woodruff, G. (1981). *Early intervention for children with special needs and their families: Findings and recommendations.* Westar Series Paper No. 11. Seattle, WA: University of Washington, 1981. ED 207 278.

Goetze, L. D. (2007, January). *Utah preschool, cost, quality, and outcomes study.* Final report prepared for the Utah State Office of Education Lead Finance Committee Meeting.

Greene, J. C., Caracelli, V. I., & Graham, W. F. (1989). Toward a conceptual framework for mixed-method evaluation designs. *Educational Evaluation and Policy Analysis, 11,* 255–274.

Grunewald, R., & Markeson, B. (2007). *Enriching children, enriching the nation: Public investment in high-quality prekindergarten*— book review summary. Retrieved from http://www.minneapolisfed.org/research/pub_display.cfm?id=1136

Gupta, D. K. (2001). *Analyzing public policy: Concepts, tools, and techniques.* Washington, DC: CQ Press.

Halpern, D. F. (1987). *Student outcomes assessment: What institutions stand to gain.* San Francisco: Jossey-Bass.

Harbin, G., Rous, B., & McLean, M. (2005). Feature article: Issues in designing state accountability systems. *Journal of Early Intervention, 27*(3), 137–164.

Hatry, H. P. & Kopczynski, M. (1997). *Guide to program outcome measurement for the U.S. Department of Education.* Washington, DC: Department of Education, Planning and Evaluation Service.

Kagan, S. L., & Scott-Little, C. (2004). Early learning standards: Changing the parlance and practice of early childhood education? *Phi Delta Kappan, 85,* 388–396.

Kaplan, S. A., & Garrett, K. E. (2005). The use of logic models by community-based initiatives. *Evaluation and Program Planning 28,* 167–172.

Killion, J. (2007). *Assessing impact: Evaluating staff development* (2nd ed.). Newbury Park, CA: Sage Publications and NSDC.

Lynch, R. (2007). *Enriching children, enriching the nation: Public investment in high quality pre-kindergarten.* Washington, DC: Economic Policy Institute.

Masse, L. N., & Barnett, W. S. (2002). *A benefit-cost analysis of the Abecedarian Early Childhood Intervention.* New Brunswick, NJ: National Institute for Early Education Research, Rutgers University.

Maude, S. P., & Corso, R. M. (2010). *STAR NET Evaluation Model 2009–2012.* Unpublished evaluation document.

Maude, S. P., & Corso, R. M. (in development). *The evolution of evaluation in a state-wide professional development system: Lessons learned.* Manuscript in preparation.

McNamara, C. (2010). Basic guide to program evaluation. Retrieved from http://managementhelp.org/evaluatn/fnl_eval.htm

Meisels, S. J. (2007). Accountability in early childhood: No easy answers. In R. C. Pianta, M. J. Cox, & K. Snow (Eds.), *School readiness, early learning and the transition to kindergarten.* Baltimore: Paul H. Brookes.

Pre-K Now. (2010). *Meeting standards.* Retrieved from http://www.preknow.org/educators/resource/meetingstandards.cfm

Raizen, S., & Rossi, P. (1981). *Program evaluation in education: When? How? To what ends?* Washington, DC: National Academy Press.

Reisman, J. (1994). *The evaluation forum: Helping organizations define and measure outcomes.* Organizational Research Services (ORS), Inc. Seattle, WA: Clegg & Associates.

Reisman, J., & Clegg, J. (2000). *Outcomes for success!* Seattle, WA: Clegg & Associates.

Reynolds, A. J., Temple, J. A., Robertson, D. L., & Mann, E. A. (2001). Long-term effects of an early childhood intervention on educational achievement and juvenile arrest: A 15-year follow-up of low-income children in public schools. *Journal of the American Medical Association, 285,* 2339–2346.

Rolnick, A. J., & Grunewald, R. (2003). *Early childhood development: Economic development with a high public return.* Minneapolis, MN: Minneapolis Federal Gazette.

Rous, B., McCormick, K., Gooden, C., & Townley, K. F. (2007). Kentucky's early childhood continuous assessment and accountability system: Local decisions and state supports. *Topics in Early Childhood Special Education, (27)*1, 19–33.

Schweinhart, L. J., Barnes, H. V., & Weikart, D. P. (1993). *Significant benefits: The HighScope Perry Preschool study through age 27* (Monographs of the HighScope Educational Research Foundation, 10). Ypsilanti, MI: HighScope Press.

Scott-Little, C, Kagan, S. L., Frelow, V. S., & Reid, J. (2009). Infant-toddler early learning guidelines: The content that states have addressed and implications for programs serving children with disabilities. *Infants and Young Children, 22* (2), 87–99.

Scriven, M. (1967). The methodology of evaluation. In R. E. Stake (Ed.), *Curriculum evaluation.* American Educational Research Association Monograph on Evaluation, No. 1. Chicago: Rand McNally.

Scriven, M. (1973). The methodology of evaluation. In B. R. Worthen & J. R. Sanders, *Educational evaluations: Theory and practice.* Belmont, CA: Wadsworth.

Stake, R. (2003). *Standards-based and responsive evaluation.* Newbury Park, CA: Sage Publications.

Stecher, B. M., & Davis, W. A. (1987). *How to focus an evaluation.* Newbury Park, CA: Sage Publications.

Trefler, D. (2009). Quality is free: A cost-benefit analysis of early child development initiatives. *Journal of Paediatrics and Child Health, 14,* 681–684.

United Way of America. (1996). *Measuring program outcomes: A practical approach.* Washington, DC: Author.

Vedung, E. (2000). *Public policy and program evaluation.* New Brunswick, NJ: Transaction Publishers.

Vermont Department of Education. (2003). *Vermont Early Learning Standards* (VELS). Montpelier, VT: Author.

W. K. Kellogg Foundation (WKKF). (2004). *Logic model development guide: Using logic models to bring together planning, evaluation, and action.* Battle Creek, MI: Author.

Weiss, C. H. (1997). *Evaluation* (2nd ed.). Alexandria, VA: Prentice Hall.

Westmoreland, H., Lopez, M. E., & Rosenberg, H. (2009, November). *How to develop a logic model for districtwide family engagement strategies.* Cambridge, MA: Harvard Family Research Project.

Wholey, J. S., Hatry, H. P., & Newcomer, K. E. (1994). *Handbook of practical program evaluation.* San Francisco: Jossey-Bass.

Worthen, B. R., & Sanders, J. R. (1987). *Educational evaluation: Alternative approaches and practical guidelines.* New York: Longman.

Chapter 8

Cost-Effectiveness and Efficacy of Programs

Kathleen Hebbeler and Donna Spiker

O ne of the changes made to the Individuals with Disabilities Education Act (IDEA) in the 2004 amendments involved a rather minor word change. The amendment indicated that the primary focus of federal and state monitoring of the law was to be on improving educational results and functional outcomes for all children with disabilities. Although this may seem like common sense, this directive to monitor results was the culmination of a gradual realization that monitoring the process aspects of IDEA alone was not enough to ensure successful outcomes for children with disabilities. IDEA has its historical roots in assuring the right to a free, appropriate public education for children with disabilities. Earlier versions of the law emphasized the importance of access to education because the law was enacted in response to children with disabilities being denied an education. After several decades of focusing on access, a national study revealed that outcomes for students who had received special education services were problematic, with high dropout rates for some groups and others not being able to live independently after secondary school (Wagner, Blackorby, Cameto, Hebbeler, & Newman, 1993). These findings alerted the nation that a focus on access was not enough. In 2002, the President's Commission on Excellence in Special Education strongly supported the need for a stronger focus on results. Their first recommendation emphasized the importance of looking at results:

> IDEA will only fulfill its intended purpose if it raises expectations for students and becomes result-oriented—not driven by process, litigation, regulation and confrontation. In short, the system must be judged by the opportunities it provides and the outcomes

achieved for each child. (President's Commission on Excellence in Special Education, 2002, p. 8)

When the 2004 amendment to IDEA codified the focus on results, it represented a minor word change, but it was a significant policy shift in what constitutes effective special education and early intervention services. The need to monitor results was accompanied in the law by strong emphasis on the use of evidence-based practices. Research has been conducted for many years to examine what works for children with disabilities. In 2004, IDEA made the use of effective practices for children with disabilities and the attainment of outcomes a matter of federal policy.

This chapter summarizes what is known and what we need to know about producing results for young children with special needs, including the costs of those services. We begin the chapter by introducing the reader to some basic terms from the literature that we will use throughout the chapter. Some of these terms, especially those related to economic analyses, are sometimes used interchangeably in discussions of programs for young children. Our goal is to provide and use commonly accepted definitions in hopes of increasing the sophistication of the discussion about costs and cost-effectiveness of services. The research on the cost savings associated with providing services to young children whose families live in poverty has been extensively presented in both the professional literature and the popular press and is often cited by advocates as part of the rationale for providing or expanding services for young children. The chapter provides a brief summary of this literature because it has played such a crucial role in the recent expansion of services for children under 5. The applicability of this research to services for young children with disabilities is limited, as will be discussed. Our discussion of costs and results for young children with disabilities addresses what we know about costs of services, efficacy and effectiveness, and cost-effectiveness. The chapter closes with a discussion of future trends and what additional information is needed to make good decisions about programs and services to improve outcomes. A critical distinction for serving children with disabilities that will be referenced throughout the chapter is the difference between research on improving child outcomes through the study of a particular intervention or practice, and data about the national system of early intervention (EI) services and early childhood special education (ECSE) services being provided to children and families under the auspices of IDEA. Research on practices and studies on the implementation of IDEA are both important, but knowing the former does not provide knowledge of the latter, and this is central to the difference between efficacy and effectiveness.

BASIC CONCEPTS

What does it cost to provide early intervention in Program A? How does this compare to the costs of Program B? Is didactic instruction more effective at promoting language than embedded interventions? What is the total cost of early childhood special education in Minnesota? What would be the cost of implementing a different service delivery model? Is providing two two-hour home visits a month more cost-effective than four one-hour visits? Is early intervention a good investment? Is it more cost-effective to serve preschoolers with disabilities in community child care or in preschools operated by their school district?

These represent just a small sample of the many important questions that can be asked about costs and outcomes for programs for young children with disabilities. They are the kind of questions that some administrators and policy makers are asking, and that many more should be asking. Families, as consumers of services, also have a right to know what interventions work and whether their child's program is effective. Teachers and therapists need to know what works so they can make informed decisions in selecting and modifying interventions. If two interventions are equally effective, then there is no justification for implementing one that costs more. Public resources for education, health, and social programs have always been scarce and almost certainly will continue to be so. Neither families nor taxpayers are well served if programs are spending more money than they need to or are not maximizing the results from the dollars being spent.

Having accurate information on the costs of programs is essential to providing effective and efficient services for young children with disabilities and their families. The goal of a *cost analysis* is to determine the economic value of all the resources used to provide the services in a given program (Escobar, Barnett, & Goetze, 1994). Identifying the full cost of EI and ECSE can be challenging because there are multiple costs to operating a program, some of which are paid for with public or private funds and others which are not. A common mistake in cost analysis is using a program's budget as a source of cost information, which will tend to miss some important costs. If a preschool program has two parent volunteers in the classroom at all times, then part of the cost of providing that program is the cost of the parents' time, even though the program may not be paying for it. Assuming the program is effective and another program wanted to replicate it, one could not ignore the hours of parent time that are a resource required to operate the program. Unpacking the costs of a program allows for a determination of the overall costs and also permits identification of who is incurring costs while providing information on the necessary support required if a program is to be transported to a new site (Hummel-Rossi & Ashdown, 2002). Other costs that may be overlooked are the costs of parents providing transportation to the program or the costs of classroom space when a preschool is housed in an elementary school. An alternative to calculating costs is to calculate expenditures, which is sometimes the only feasible option (see e.g., Erickson, 1992). *Expenditures* refer to resources that the program expends.

Many cost analyses use a resource cost model that involves estimating costs for all of the program's resources. This approach requires a complete description of all of the program's components, including personnel, supplies, materials, equipment, transportation, and facilities. Other resources such as using volunteers and parent time must also be included in the costs (Chambers & Parrish, 1994; Levin, 1983; Levin & McEwan, 2000). The first step in this approach involves identifying all of the program activities or ingredients, and the second step is to determine the cost of each one (Barnett, 2000).

Another issue related to costs is the identification of the *funding sources* the programs draws on. Both EI and ECSE, for example, are supported by a variety of funding sources, including a variety of federal funds along with state funds and, in some places, local funds. Another possible funding source for early intervention is private insurance and parent fees. IDEA allows states to charge parents for early intervention services, which is a funding option with both strengths and weaknesses (Mackey-Andrews & Taylor, 2007).

Both cost-benefit analyses and cost-effectiveness analyses are intended to present information to assist in decision-making. A *cost-benefit* or benefit-cost analysis (the terms are used interchangeably) refers to an analysis of the resources used and the results produced by a program or policy. In a cost-benefit analysis, monetary values are estimated for both the resources used (which are the costs) and the results produced (the benefits). A cost-benefit analysis considers the benefits and costs to both the government and to society. The goal is to provide information about whether the programs, services, and practices are paying off economically: are there lasting positive outcomes for children and their families, and do the savings outweigh the costs? (National Research Council and Institute of Medicine, 2009). One of the challenges in cost-benefit analysis is the difficulty in assigning monetary value to some of the outcomes (Barnett, 2000). For example, assigning a dollar value to an increase in parenting confidence produced by an early intervention program will be difficult. *Cost-effectiveness analysis* differs from a benefit-cost analysis in that a dollar value is not placed on the outcome in a cost-effectiveness outcome. The costs and outcomes of one intervention or service can be compared with the costs and outcomes of another treatment. The results of the analysis are reported in terms of how much must be invested to achieve a given level of the outcome (National Research Council and Institute of Medicine, 2009). For example, a cost-effectiveness analysis could identify the cost associated with improving a preschooler's communication skills by five standard scores points on a developmental assessment using a particular intervention. A cost-effectiveness analysis allows a comparison of the relative costs of different approaches required to reach the same level of outcome or of the relative level of outcomes achieved by different interventions with the same costs.

Cost-effectiveness studies require two distinct kinds of information: information on costs, and information on outcomes. Research makes a distinction between two kinds of studies that look at outcomes. *Efficacy studies* examine whether or not interventions, practices, or programs can work in the ideal, highly controlled situation in which interventions are implemented as intended by practitioners or researchers who have been highly trained in the procedures. *Effectiveness* studies are designed to look at interventions in real-life situations and address whether the intervention works when it is implemented in programs as they operate in day-to-day life (Blackman, 2000). Not surprisingly, interventions shown to be efficacious may not turn out to be effective because, for example, they are too difficult or cumbersome for practitioners to implement faithfully. Both kinds of studies are important to understanding and promoting improved outcomes for children and families. Cost-effectiveness analysis can use data from either efficacy or effectiveness studies depending on whether the outcome data is collected from a controlled implementation or implementation in real-world programs.

ECONOMIC ANALYSES OF PROGRAMS FOR YOUNG CHILDREN AT ENVIRONMENTAL RISK

In 1999, the National Academy of Sciences convened a national panel to consider the science behind the notion that the early years of life are critical in laying the foundation for the optimal development of our nation's children. In reviewing the extensive research about early childhood development in the neurobiological, behavioral, and social sciences (National Research Council and Institute of Medicine, 2000), the panel concluded that the early years are indeed critical for setting the stage for long-term favorable or unfavorable developmental outcomes of all children. Furthermore, they concluded that much can be done to increase the chances that more children will experience favorable outcomes.

Several of the panel's recommendations were in response to the well-documented and unfortunate reality that young children exposed to environmental risk, most notably poverty, are likely to acquire new skills and behaviors at a much slower rate than their more advantaged peers in the years leading up to kindergarten (Hart & Risley, 1995; Lee & Burkam, 2002). In turn, poor school readiness at kindergarten entry has been shown to lead to long-term consequences including poor school achievement. New research on the importance of the early years for brain development combined with the significant achievement gap at kindergarten entry for children from low-income families has resulted in substantial interest in policies and programs to address this problem. A sizable body of research has shown that high-quality ECE programs can be successful in promoting school readiness of young children, particularly those living in low-income families (Karoly et al., 1998). Programs for children at risk of poor developmental outcomes have been heavily promoted to policy makers by presenting a body of research demonstrating the costs and benefits of early childhood programs, services, and practices (Barnett, 2000; Karoly & Bigelow, 2005; Karoly et al., 1998; Karoly, Kilburn, Bigelow, Caulkins, & Cannon, 2001; National Research Council and Institute of Medicine, 2009). Providing programs to address the developmental needs of young children living in poverty is not a new idea; Head Start, for example, was created in the 1960s based on the existing evidence of poor school performance for children in poverty. The rationale for providing programs to address this problem was significantly strengthened with the new research on brain development and the very conclusive evidence that the long-term benefits of such programs far outweigh the costs.

In particular, policy makers have been impressed by cost-benefit data from three model programs—the Perry Preschool Program, the Abecedarian Project, and the Chicago Child-Parent Centers. Research on these programs indicates significant short- and long-term benefits that include increased school achievement and educational attainment, reduced juvenile delinquency and criminality, and better adult workforce participation (Karoly et al., 1998). Longitudinal outcomes studies that followed program participants into adulthood indicate that the benefits calculated outweigh program costs while boosting long-term academic, social, and occupational achievement, particularly for children from low-income families who are at greatest risk for poor school readiness and subsequent school failure (Barnett & Masse, 2007; Heckman & Masterov, 2004; Karoly & Bigelow, 2005; Reynolds, Temple, Robertson, & Mann, 2002; Schweinhart, 2004). Across cost-benefit studies of high-quality preschool programs for children with low-income families, the cost savings estimates have ranged from just under $3 up to $17 for every dollar spent (Barnett & Masse, 2007; Belfield, Nores, Barnett, & Schweinhart, 2006; Schweinhart et al., 2005; Temple & Reynolds, 2007).

Such cost-benefit findings have led states all over the country to increase their investments in state-funded preschool programs, even with huge state budget deficits (Gallagher, Clayton, & Heinemeier, 2001; Kauerz, 2001; National Governors Association, 2005). In an influential report, Karoly (2005) estimated that California would receive $2.7 billion in present value net benefits for implementing high-quality, one-year voluntary universal preschool attended by 70 percent of eligible 4-year-olds (i.e., for every dollar spent on preschool programs, there would be a savings of $2.62).

Despite the prominence of a small set of cost-benefit analyses and the growing support for the importance of early childhood programs, very few program models have actually been subjected to a cost-benefit analysis (Karoly, Kilburn, & Cannon, 2005). Cost savings may be far less for less well-resourced program models. The programs that produced the impressive benefits and cost savings were very well implemented, comprehensive, intensive programs with highly trained staff. Not all preschool programs match the level of quality in these model programs. Accordingly, the magnitude of the benefits has not been as large for other preschool programs such as Head Start and state-funded preschool programs (Howes et al., 2008; Zill et al., 2003). Nevertheless, preschool programs judged to have high-quality instruction have been shown to yield positive impacts on low-income children's school readiness in cognitive, language, and social skills (Anderson et al., 2003; Barnett & Hustedt, 2005; Currie & Thomas, 1995).

We have presented a brief overview of the findings from this select set of cost-benefit studies because they have had a significant impact on early childhood policy in the last decade. The findings tend to be cited to justify many different kinds of investments in programs for young children. It is important to remember that these programs were implemented with young children in poverty, and that is the only population to which the findings apply. These programs were not designed to address the needs of children with disabilities, nor were they implemented with this population. It is interesting that children with disabilities have certainly benefitted from this body of work because it has helped alert policy makers to the importance of a child's early years, and also because it has resulted in an increase in preschool programs providing more options for inclusive settings for preschoolers with disabilities.

One can reasonably maintain that these programs did indeed prevent developmental delay by significantly improving the development and learning of children who were already or were on their way to being very low functioning. Some researchers maintain that the children in the Perry Preschool Project met the criteria for mental retardation, and even though these children might not have received that diagnosis today with more sophisticated assessment procedures, the data do suggest the children were fairly low functioning with regard to intellectual development (Barnett & Escobar, 1988). Children with developmental delays, however, make up only one segment of the population of children with disabilities. We cannot conclude that programs for children with disabilities would return the same kind of economic benefits because programs for children from low-income families show such benefits. To reach conclusions about the benefits and cost-effectiveness of programs for children with disabilities, we need to look to the research on programs and interventions designed for this population.

COSTS OF PROVIDING SERVICES TO YOUNG CHILDREN WITH DISABILITIES

Widespread agreement exists about both the need for and challenges associated with obtaining good data on the cost of programs for young children with disabilities (Macy & Schafer, 1985; Roberts, Innocenti, & Goetze, 1999; Tarr & Barnett, 2001). Some past studies have relied on budgets that provide incomplete data on the full cost of services (Barnett & Escobar, 2002). Other challenges include the diversity in the children served and the diversity in the programs themselves. Neither early intervention nor early childhood special education is a well-defined program model. Rather, each is a collection of services delivered in different ways, in different settings, by different professionals at individually determined intensities. How programs are staffed and stuctured varies across the country, making it difficult to generalize cost findings from one locality or state to another. Finally, cost analyses that focus on producing a total per-program cost or a per-child cost may become dated very quickly as costs change with inflation or programmatic changes. All of these challenges have probably contributed to having very few studies on the costs of serving young children with disabilities.

Cost analyses can produce the total cost to operate a program, or costs to serve a particular type of child, or both. An interesting analysis of total cost was completed by Chambers (1991) to assist California in projecting the costs to the state of participating in Part C (then referred to as Part H). The analysis made projections about the number of children likely to be identified and calculated service costs, along with costs for all the program components such as the development of the IFSP, outreach and public awareness, and the cost of the Interagency Coordinating Council. In the spirit of a cost-benefit analysis, Chambers noted that the state needed to consider whether the costs are outweighed by the long-term benefits of providing services to this population.

A study in Massachusetts based on data from 1988 calculated the hourly cost of various kinds of services. The study found that home visits cost $53.68 per hour; a center-based individual session, $45.28 per hour; a child-focused group session, $21.52 per hour; and a parent support group session, $14.72 per hour (Warfield, 1994). Escobar et al. (1994) calculated costs for 11 home-based and center-based early intervention programs in seven states. In 1990 dollars, the range in costs for the home-based programs was from $3,617 to $7,693 per child, and the range for the center-based programs was from $3,228 to $14,123. Across programs, personnel costs ranged from 35 to 65 percent of total program costs. An analysis of early intervention in New Jersey in 1996 found an average cost of $7,933 per year per IFSP with substantial variation across programs (Tarr & Barnett, 2001). The authors note that at time the data were collected, the state was providing center-based services and that shortly thereafter, the state had begun serving more children and families in natural environments, an example of a programmatic change with a high likelihood of impacting costs.

The only national data on the cost of early intervention comes from the National Early Intervention Longitudinal Study (NEILS). This study followed a nationally representative sample from the time they began early intervention in 1997 or 1998 until the end of their kindergarten year. Applying a resource-cost-model approach to data for a subsample of 2,195 children with adequate service data, the study calculated per-child expenditures for the child's total time in early intervention. The estimates were expenditures for services received from the initial IFSP through program exit, did not include costs for service coordination, and represented only the agencies' cost, not any costs incurred by the family. The average total spending for the average total stay in early intervention of 17.2 months was estimated to be $15,740 per child or $916 per month (Hebbeler, Levin, Perez, Lam, & Chambers, 2009; Levin, Perez, Lam, Chambers, & Hebbeler, 2004).

Cost analyses also look at how costs differ for different groups or what explains variation in costs. NEILS found substantial variation in expenditure for children with different disabilities. Monthly expenditures for children with risk conditions were $549; for children with only communication delays, $642; for children with developmental delay, $948; and for children with diagnosed conditions, $1,103. NEILS also found substantial variation within these groups. For example, for children with developmental delays, the median expenditure was $588 (compared to a mean of $948), the 25th percentile was $282, and the 75th was $1,128 (Hebbeler et al., 2009). Looking at variation across EI programs, Tarr & Barnett (2001) found that programs where staff spent a greater proportion of time in direct service delivery had lower costs. Programs with more aides had lower costs as did programs where more time was spent delivering services in a group. Escobar et al. (1994), in their study of 11 programs, found that the factors with the greatest impact on costs were program duration and frequency of service (measured in hours per year), intensity of service, geographic location, and contributed resources.

Other cost analyses for services for young children with disabilities have examined costs of particular models or practices Odom and his colleagues (2001) studied the costs of preschool inclusion by comparing instructional costs (not total costs) of community-based and Head Start–inclusive programs with the costs of more traditional preschool special education classrooms. Across the 14 programs in 5 states, there were 9 possible within local education agency (LEA) comparisons of inclusive to traditional programs. In six of the nine comparisons, the inclusive programs were less expensive than the traditional program. Costs to the LEA ranged from $1,576 to $4,963 for the traditional programs, and from $941 to $6,886 for the inclusive programs.

Studies such as these, although relatively rare, provide a foundation for understanding what it costs to provide services and what are some of the factors that lead services to go up or down. Far more information would be helpful, particularly related to the implementation of early intervention and early childhood special education across the country. More information on cost would be helpful as new practices or program models are being developed, so potential adopters could make more informed decisions.

RESEARCH ON THE EFFICACY AND EFFECTIVENESS OF EI AND ECSE

There is a clear need for continuing to expand the knowledge base on interventions and practices to promote good outcomes for young children with disabilities, and we need to know more about what works, for whom, and under what circumstances (Guralnick, 1989, 2005b). However, there is actually a fairly large body of research on the efficacy and effectiveness of early intervention (EI) and early childhood special education (ECSE) that has grown steadily over the past five decades (Guralnick, 1997, 2005b; Shonkoff & Meisels, 2000). To understand efficacy research, it is important to understand what EI and ECSE are trying to do. The goals of these programs have remained the same: (1) to promote and advance the development and skills of infants, toddlers, and preschoolers, and (2) to support and assist families in promoting the development and skills of infants, toddlers, and preschoolers. The outcomes for children have become broader and more functional (Spiker, Hebbeler, & Mallik, 2005). Parents, practitioners, and researchers agree that EI and ECSE services help to lay a foundation for the child's lifelong learning. This foundation is expected to help the child achieve higher levels of functioning that will support full participation in family, school, and community life, and lead to a good quality of life. Similarly, EI and ECSE provide a foundation for the family to be able to help the child learn and grow; participate fully in family, school, and community; and have a good quality of life *as a family*. It is also important to note that as recently as the 1970s, children with disabilities were institutionalized based on low expectations about their ability to participate in home, school, and community life. Such low expectations and the tremendous costs of institutionalization were unfortunate, and they also served to limit educational policies, available services and programs, and the kind of research that was funded and conducted. IDEA changed the landscape of education for children with disabilities, including infants, toddlers, and preschoolers. The law raised expectations for what children could achieve and also increased the importance of using effective practices in the service of promoting good outcomes.

Given the changing historical landscape, what does the research tell us about the effectiveness of EI and ECSE for infants, toddlers, and preschoolers with disabilities? Understanding the efficacy research on programs or services for young children with disabilities requires appreciating the implications of three characteristics of this population and the programs provided. First, EI and ECSE consist of a wide range of services. These services range from special instruction for the child to therapies (e.g., physical, occupational, speech), family training, and a variety of specialized services (e.g., audiology, vision or assistive technology services, diagnosis and evaluation) that are delivered in a variety of settings by many different kinds of professionals and paraprofessionals (Guralnick, 1997, 2005b; Hebbeler, Barton, & Mallik, 2008; Hebbeler, Spiker, Morrison, & Mallik, 2008; Spiker & Hebbeler, 1999). As will be described below, some studies have focused on the effects of receiving or not receiving a specific type of service (e.g., physical therapy). Most efficacy studies are about specific practices or strategies to promote children's learning or development.

Second, there is considerable variability among young children with disabilities with regard to their types of disabilities; the severity of their delays and functioning levels; their rates of skill acquisition; their health status and conditions; social, behavioral and temperamental characteristics; and ultimately, their developmental and educational outcomes (Scarborough et al., 2004; Scarborough, Hebbeler, & Spiker, 2006) and chapters on specific disabilities in Guralnick (1997). Many studies focus on effectiveness of a practice or intervention for children with specific types of disabilities.

Third, related to this child variability, EI and ECSE services are by design expected to be individualized to address the very different needs and functioning levels of the children served. Children receive different constellations of services, with different intensity over differing durations. Even when the service is ostensibly the same, providers will implement adaptations when providing services that accommodate the needs of the particular children (e.g., different children with gross motor delays receive physical therapy, but the characteristics of the therapy will vary to meet the child's specific needs). The implication of the diversity of the children, the diversity of the services, and individualization based on need is that much of what we know about the efficacy of practices or interventions under circumscribed conditions has not been tested in the full range of programs and populations that make up EI and ECSE in the "real world."

Overview of Efficacy Studies with Young Children with Disabilities

Efficacy research has demonstrated many benefits of intervention for infants, toddlers, and preschoolers with disabilities (Bailey et al., 2006; Guralnick, 1997, 2001, 2005b; Spiker, Hebbeler, & Mallik, 2005) that include the following:

- Acceleration of skills and behaviors that eliminates delay and leads to normal functioning
- Acceleration of skill acquisition and improved functioning that improves the child's developmental trajectory without attaining normal functioning
- Prevention of abnormal patterns or functioning that would lead to greater delay and dysfunction
- Promotion of optimal parent-child interactions that facilitate the child's development and functioning
- Provision of helpful parent support to allow parents to better facilitate the child's development and functioning
- Encouragement of the child's participation in inclusive settings

Some of the earliest EI and ECSE programs were research demonstration projects in the 1960s, 1970s, and 1980s. These early programs tended to be broad-based parent training and center-based programs that focused on promoting cognitive, language, communication, and motor skills. "Training" strategies were used that emphasized stimulus-response learning models and behavior modification strategies, with the parents being trained to "stimulate" the child. These studies showed benefits of these programs compared with control groups in the United States, England, Canada, and Australia (Farran, 1990;

Farran, 2000; Gibson & Harris, 1988; Guralnick & Bricker, 1987; Spiker & Hopmann, 1997). The results showed increased rates of development of skills and milestones and slower declines in the rate of development as measured by global developmental or IQ tests. It is worth noting that these and many subsequent efficacy studies actually test the effect of specific practices, strategies, or program models for teaching children or assisting parents to help them learn rather than testing the impact of a type of service per se (e.g., speech therapy).

By the 1990s, a body of research on interventions for this population showed benefits for both children and families (Guralnick, 1997; Spiker & Hopmann, 1997). IDEA had created a national program for early intervention and for early childhood special education and service provision had moved toward individual intervention plans that involved a combination of services and supports. A recent review (Spiker, Hebbeler, & Mallik, 2005) noted that the "constellation of services and supports might include:

- Information about the child's disability
- Ongoing health monitoring to meet both routine and specialized medical needs
- Individualized one-to-one services and therapies targeted to promote specific skill acquisition and improvements in functioning
- Parent education and training focused on optimal responsivity to promote the child's learning and participation in daily activities and routines
- Opportunities for interactions with peers in group settings" (p. 316–317).

The research documenting benefits of these kinds of services and supports have been extensively reviewed, including reviews that focus on specific types of disabilities (Guralnick, 1997, 2005b; Lord et al., 2005; Shonkoff & Meisels, 2000). Here again, many of the more recent studies document the effectiveness of specific interventions or services for specific outcomes or children (e.g., physical therapy for children with motor delays), or applied behavior analysis (ABA) teaching methods (described below), or strategies for promoting optimal parent-child interactions by providing parents with information about children's specific disability or delay and early development, by modeling of stimulating interactions, and by providing positive emotional support (Dunst, Trivette, & Jodry, 1997; Kelly, Booth-LaForce, & Spiker, 2005; Spiker, Boyce, & Boyce, 2002). Implementing rigorous study designs (e.g., randomized trials) for a population for whom individualized services are required by law raises many challenges, and even studies with random assignment using a treatment-as-usual control group are logistically difficult to implement fully when knowledgeable parents seek out potentially beneficial treatments and researchers cannot control treatment switching (described by Lord et al. [2005] in treatment studies about autism).

Four common areas of research are summarized briefly in the next sections to illustrate the types of efficacy studies that have been done.

Efficacy of Applied Behavior Analysis

The earliest studies from the 1960s to the 1980s mainly examined effects of behavior modification or stimulus-response approaches, also known as applied behavior analysis (ABA; Gardner, 2006). ABA has been extensively researched, with many studies showing how ABA techniques can help establish behaviors as well as consolidate and generalize them, using reinforcement principles and stimulus-response models of learning (Cooper, Heron, & Heward, 2007). These kinds of studies were highly controlled investigations of specific practices, not a type of service or a program. Many of these early efficacy studies focused on discrete behaviors of individuals that often were decontextualized, and these results have been criticized for leading to skills learned in this way did not generalize and were not easily used by the child in everyday situations.

More recent ABA approaches that have been the focus of efficacy studies involve more contextualized learning and focus on more meaningful behaviors such as errorless learning, chaining, functional analysis, naturalistic teaching, and pivotal response training (Koegel & Koegel, 2006). For instance, pivotal response training, particularly developed for use with young children with autism but applicable to all young children with disabilities, aims to intentionally teach children key behaviors that help them "learn to learn," emphasizing a child's motivation to learn by explicitly teaching behaviors relevant for initiating and maintaining social interactions, using joint attention skills, being responsive to multiple cues, and learning other attention and self-regulation behaviors (Koegel & Koegel, 2006). This and other recent naturalistic learning approaches (1) emphasize teaching functional behaviors in natural settings rather than using isolated, rote learning approaches; (2) have a large and growing research base to support their efficacy for promoting children's early academic, language, and social skills; and (3) have as an explicit goal supporting the inclusion of young children with disabilities in settings with typical peers (Wolery, 2000). It is also noteworthy that many of the ABA studies focused on a single type of disability, such as autism; many focus on a specific curriculum; and some practices are supported by single subject study designs.

Efficacy of Interventions with Parents

Strategies for working with parents have been the focus of many studies because it is well recognized that the amount of time that children actually receive a professionally delivered intervention is small compared to the amount of time and the number of learning opportunities that parents have with their young children. As described above, some of the early EI and ECSE programs were parent training programs, teaching parents how to apply ABA methods with their children (at the time referred to as behavior modification; reviewed by Spiker & Hopmann, 1997). Based on a large body of basic research about how children's earliest interactions with adults provide the basis for their language acquisition and cognitive development, more recent studies show positive impacts of parent-child interaction intervention models to promote children's language, communication, and cognitive development (Mahoney & Perales, 2005; Roper & Dunst, 2003; Warren, 2000; Yoder & Warren, 2004). A review of effectiveness studies concluded that there is strong evidence that highly responsive adult-child interactions promote language acquisition and learning (Mahoney, Boyce, Fewell, Spiker, & Wheeden, 1998). Parent training studies also showing the effectiveness of strategies to help parents learn effective ways to handle and manage children's behavior to prevent or remediate behavior problems that interfere with learning (Webster-Stratton, 1997).

Efficacy Studies about Practices for Promoting Language, Communication, and Social Development

Because language and communication delays and difficulties are common across most young children with disabilities, and these skills are essential for school and life success and to promote the goal of full participation (inclusion), practices and strategies to address them have been the subject of a great number of studies. The earliest studies examining how to promote speech and communication skills tended to focus on interventions to teach children sounds, words, etc., and use operant or stimulus-response training methods. Recent advances in understanding of prelinguistic and language and communication acquisition have led the field away from using decontextualized, non-functional approaches for teaching and supporting young children's communication skills. The rich research base about prelinguistic communication with infants and toddlers has emerged relatively recently. Research also has demonstrated that the amount and quality of language input are important for children's language development (Hart & Risley, 1995). Furthermore, the movement toward inclusion in settings with typical peers gives children with disabilities opportunities for peer interactions that are beneficial to acquiring and using language. Drawing on this basic developmental research, newer studies have demonstrated the positive impact of strategies that support highly responsive and functional conversations, both with peers and adults, in natural contexts in promoting children's communication and cognitive skills (McCathren, Yoder, & Warren, 1995; Roper & Dunst, 2003) Many of the findings from parent-child interaction interventions (described above) are relevant to how teachers interact with young children in classroom settings.

Efficacy Studies about Inclusive Educational Programming

Many recent studies have looked how to promote participation of young children with disabilities in inclusive settings (Guralnick, 2001, 2005b). The inclusion of children with disabilities in programs that serve typically developing children is perhaps the most remarkable change in education over the past several decades—brought about by parent advocacy and a legislative requirement that children with disabilities are to be educated in the least restrictive environment (DEC/NAEYC, 2009; Fuchs & Fuchs, 1994). Inclusion gives young children with disabilities access to the general early childhood curriculum, typical peers, and more of the typical activities available to other children, holding a promise of achieving better child outcomes.

Beginning in the 1980s, experimental inclusion programs began to demonstrate that it was possible to offer inclusive programs and that children with disabilities could make good progress in them (Bricker, 2000; Guralnick, 2005a). By the 1990s, some research was demonstrating how inclusive early childhood programs could be implemented successfully (e.g., Wolery & Wilbers, 1994). A review of 22 studies found that preschool-age children with disabilities have better outcomes on standard measures of development, social competence, play behavior, and engagement when served in inclusive rather than segregated settings (Buysse & Bailey, 1993). These findings are supported by more recent data as well (Guralnick, 2001). Others have argued that the evidence base for the efficacy of inclusive programs to produce good child outcomes is still relatively meager, although the practice has proliferated (Bricker, 2000). Responding to the myriad of definitions of inclusion in the research literature, a recently released joint position statement by the Division for Early Childhood and the National Association for the Education of Young Children (DEC/ NAEYC, 2009) defines inclusion as consisting of (1) access, i.e., a wide range of typical environments and use of universal design to support full access; (2) participation, i.e., suggested approaches to support and promote the child's full participation, such as embedded instructional approaches; and (3) supports, i.e., infrastructure to support staff, such as appropriate professional development opportunities and specialized services in the setting. Currently, many infants, toddlers, and preschoolers with disabilities participate in a wide range of early care and education programs, some of which also serve typically developing children (e.g., center-based and family-based child care, Head Start, state-funded preschool programs) and some of which serve children with disabilities exclusively (e.g., school-based preschool special education programs). More research is needed about the effectiveness of any of these kinds of programs to improve child outcomes over the short and long term. A recent research study showed that a significant number of children with mild developmental delays who were fully included in preschool and kindergarten were not in an inclusive placement by first and second grade (Guralnick, Neville, Hammond, & Connor, 2008).

Implications of Efficacy and Effectiveness Studies for Cost-Effectiveness Research

This brief review suggests that at a general level, we know a great deal about how to intervene to change the developmental trajectories of young children with delays and disabilities. There is still much to be learned about tailoring interventions or practices to particular types of children or to particular settings with an as yet unknown level of intensity. Much of what is known focuses on specific services or practices, often studied with specific populations. Other studies yield child outcome data based on one feature of the program (e.g., receiving services in an inclusive preschool program). We have a strong theory for developing new interventions and a good overall picture of what works but that still needs more evidence about the application to the full range of children with delays and disabilities. Furthermore, much of the research is focused on a practice or intervention strategy, not a complete program model.

A critical and as yet unanswered question is the extent to which what we have learned from efficacy studies is reflected in the implementation of EI and ECSE programs around the country. The types of interventions, services, or practices that have been studied represent experiences that children *may* have in the real world (Hemmeter, 2000), but we do not know the extent to which children are actually having them. Many findings are based on highly controlled experimental or quasi-experimental studies that show what *can* work under ideal conditions. More research is needed to learn how typical practitioners implement evidence-based practices in a typical program and the kind of outcomes achieved in these circumstances. As described earlier, EI/ECSE is not a singular "program" in the sense that it is one consistent set of interventions that can be described with precision so they are replicable. In addition, children receive combinations of services that can vary considerably across groups of children, making it hard to define and therefore study the "treatment." Finally, different levels of outcomes attainment are appropriate for different populations (e.g., what can be expected for children with mild versus severe delays in functioning). Taking these differences into account in any cost-benefit analysis is necessary and reasonable, and similar to cost-benefit analysis in medicine, which takes into account the types and severity of a condition when examining costs of health care and health outcomes (Murray, Evans, Acharya, & Baltussen, 2000).

LOOKING AT THE COSTS AND OUTCOMES OF SERVICES FOR YOUNG CHILDREN WITH SPECIAL NEEDS

Data on costs of services is interesting, but these data alone provide limited information for decision making in policy or practice (Barnett & Escobar, 2002). Similarly, identifying and implementing effective practices and program models is critical for making short- and long-term differences in children's lives. The true power in designing effective programs comes from combining information on costs with information on effective practices so that resources can be allocated wisely.

The need for research on cost-effectiveness is widely acknowledged and has been for many years. In 1984, Senator Orrin Hatch wrote about the limited resources and difficult decisions that must be made in serving young children with disabilities. He asserted that cost-effectiveness must be a criterion in deciding how best to serve these children (Hatch, 1984). "Is the system cost-effective for the type and level of early intervention services provided for the eligible population?" was one of the key questions for Part C implementation identified by a group of evaluation professionals (Roberts et al., 1999). It is hard to argue with the importance of implementing cost-effective services. Unfortunately, the research relating costs to outcomes of programs or practices for children with disabilities is relatively sparse, and much of it is dated or not methodologically sound. Our knowledge about what works has been advancing; our knowledge of what works at what cost remains rather primitive.

One of the largest reviews of cost-effectiveness studies in EI and ECSE was conducted by Barnett and Escobar (1988). They reviewed 15 early studies of cost-benefit or cost-effectiveness of programs for young children with disabilities and found significant methodological flaws in nearly all of them, including omitting important elements from the cost analysis. They concluded their review by noting that the existing evidence provided a weak basis for making decisions on economic grounds about early intervention and called for methodologically stronger studies that follow standard economic analysis procedures.

One of these early studies compared the cost and outcomes of half-day and full-day programs for matched pairs of children in seven half-day and eight full-day classrooms (Taylor, White, & Pezzino, 1984). The study concluded that half-day programs were more cost-effective for children with cognitive impairments, and that full-day programs were more cost-effective for children with communication impairments. Conclusions about the effectiveness of the classroom were based on the performance of two children in each classroom, and no information was collected about the quality of the instruction or the qualification of the personnel in any of the classrooms. In addition, as noted by Barnett and Escobar (1988), the length of day was confounded with other program differences, and the study drew conclusions based on differences that were not statistically significant and were too small to be meaningful.

A few published studies have compared the costs of two specific services for specific types of children. In a prospective randomized trial comparing a large group community-based parent training program versus a clinic-based individual parent training program for children with disruptive behavior problems, better child behavioral outcomes were found for the community-based program. A cost analysis with matched groups of 18 participating families found the community-based intervention was more than six times as cost effective as the clinic-based treatment (Cunningham, Bremner, & Boyle, 1995). Likewise, another study that compared costs and outcomes of parent training versus clinic-based treatment for preschoolers with speech delays found no difference on costs (when parent time was excluded from the cost analysis), but the parent training program resulted in better child outcomes (Eiserman, McCoun, & Escobar, 1996).

A study conducted by Taylor, White, & Kusmierek (1993) in the late 1980s provides a good example of the challenges in conducting good cost-effectiveness research on important program features with this population. This study used random assignment to examine the benefits of more intensive early intervention services. One group was assigned to the typical EI program of one hour a week, and the experimental groups were assigned to three hours of service a week for 24 weeks. Not surprisingly, the three-hour program cost nearly three times as much as the usual program of one hour per week. The researchers collected data verifying the comparability of the two groups of children (although they did not provide information on their disabilities). They also videotaped treatment sessions, from which they determined that the interventions being provided represented best practice. The study found no difference in child outcomes across the two levels of intensity. Although this study was carefully executed from a methodological perspective, the design is inconsistent with the principle of individualized services. What went on during the session might have met the standard of best practice, but assigning all families the same amount of service would not be considered best practice. It is quite possible that in both the experimental and control groups, some families were receiving more or less service than they needed. Randomly assigning families to an arbitrary amount of service bears no resemblance to actual practice, so the findings are of limited utility to early intervention as it is practiced in the real world.

The rise in the number of young children being diagnosed with autism or autism spectrum disorders and the high cost of some intervention approaches has led to a few recent studies examining the costs of providing services to this population. For instance, a recent analysis of data from Texas estimated that providing an average of three years of intensive discrete trial training to preschoolers with autism would save about $208,000 per child when compared with the costs of 18 years of special education (Chasson, Harris, & Neely, 2007). Using data from Pennsylvania, the costs of three years of intensive behavioral treatments for children with autism between ages 2 and 5 were estimated to be between $33,000 and $50,000 per year (Jacobson, Mulick, & Green, 1998). These same researchers went on to do a cost-benefit analysis in which they assumed that 40–50 percent of the treated children achieved normal functioning by school entry, based on one widely cited randomized study (Lovaas, 1987). Their analysis estimated that the lifetime cost savings would range from about $650,000 to about $1 million per child.

Some cost-effectiveness work has been carried out on methods of identifying children in need of special services. Cost-effectiveness data and arguments have been put forward to support investments in early and periodic developmental screening (American Academy of Pediatrics Committee on Children with Disabilities, 2001; Squires, Nickels, & Eisart, 1996). Most available data addresses actual costs of developmental screenings, but are limited in showing cost benefits (Dobrez et al., 2001; Glascoe, Foster, & Wolraich, 1997). As with any type of screening service, the rationale is that by identifying a condition earlier, it can be effectively treated, thus saving the future costs associated with the condition (Murray et al., 2000). For children with mild delays detected early, the expected benefit of developmental screening is earlier access to beneficial early intervention services, which in turn will prevent the development of more significant delays or disabilities, lead to a much improved or even typical developmental trajectory prior to entering kindergarten, and avoid the increased costs associated with special education. For children with more significant delays, early detection and service receipt is considered to prevent the development of even more significant delays and give these children and their families the specialized assistance needed to maximize their development (Farran, 1990; 2000).

An example of a cost-effectiveness study of identification methods compared the costs and results of four methods of identifying developmental problems in young children (Glascoe, Foster, & Wolraich, 1997). They estimated the costs for each of the methods, collected data on how successful each was in correctly identifying children with problems, and then projected out the long-term savings associated with each method. They concluded that none of the methods was superior with regard to long-term benefits, but that the use of a two-item questionnaire to identify parents' concerns was far less costly because it required less time for physicians to administer and interpret. As the researchers point out, this kind of analysis requires making many assumptions, especially around the percentage of children who will have a given level of disability, future outcomes such as high school graduation rates for certain populations with disabilities, and whether they will require group homes as adults. Verifying that a less expensive screening method is no less effective than a more costly approach for the short-term outcome of detection of developmental problems rests on far fewer assumptions.

As with developmental screening, cost-effectiveness arguments have been made for newborn and periodic hearing screening, but with limited actual cost-benefit data (Mehl & Thomson, 1998). Early detection of hearing impairment or deafness should lead to referral to appropriate EI services, and earlier treatments with assistive devices, which in turn should promote more optimal language acquisition (Yoshinaga-Itano, 2004). Because early childhood is a critical period for language acquisition, it is predicted that anything that promotes a more typical early language acquisition trajectory will have beneficial effects on preventing subsequent school failure and later poor occupational performance. Especially with universal newborn screening, however, the limited available data are mixed in supporting arguments of lifetime cost savings, partly because severe and profound deafness detected in the newborn period is such a low-incidence condition, and many infants later identified with a congenital moderate-to-severe hearing loss actually were born with normal hearing and progressed to have hearing loss in early infancy (Karen, Helfand, Homer, McPhillips, & Lieu, 2002; Mehl & Thomson, 1998; Yoshinaga-Itano, 2004). Two studies of newborn-hearing screening have reported cost savings for the procedure. Mehl and Thomson (1998) used data on nearly 42,000 newborns screened in Colorado to conclude that all costs associated with newborn hearing screening would be recovered by the state after 10 years. Using a hypothetical birth cohort of 80,000 infants and data assembled from many different sources, Karen et al. (2002) concluded that newborn hearing screening was more cost-effective than no screening or selective screening because it resulted in better outcomes and reduced costs. As these authors note, better evidence is needed because studies have not yet quantified the true impact of early intervention on language production and subsequent productivity. Screening high-risk newborns in neonatal intensive care units (NICUs) has been suggested as a more cost-effective approach given the greater chance of secondary disability for this population (Yoshinaga-Itano, 2004). A stronger cost-benefit case has been made for periodic hearing screening throughout early childhood to detect conductive hearing losses that can usually be completely corrected and for which EI services can set the child back on a normal developmental trajectory for language development (Yoshinaga-Itano, 2004).

RECENT DEVELOPMENTS WITH IMPLICATIONS FOR STUDYING COST-EFFECTIVENESS

The review of information on cost-effectiveness for services for young children with disabilities indicates that there is much more we need to know. New contributions to the knowledge base may come in the future from state agencies. The last several years have seen substantial growth in state capacity to report data on outcomes for young children with disabilities. Spurred by a requirement from the federal government, all states have undertaken to implement statewide procedures for measuring the progress of children who receive EI or ECSE services. This development has occurred independently of, but simultaneously with, strong federal support for building longitudinal data systems in states to track children's progress across time, and some states are opting to include early childhood programs in their databases. The combination of these two forces has the potential to produce an ongoing source of data on child outcomes and, in states with sophisticated data systems, cost of these services as well, which sets the stage for future cost-effectiveness analyses.

As part of ongoing accountability, the federal government requires data on outcomes for all federally funded programs. Not unique to the federal government, the importance of promoting and monitoring outcomes is widely recognized across a variety of public and private funding sources (Hogan, 2001; Morley, Vinson, & Hatry, 2000). Since the early 1990s, all federal programs have been required by the Government Performance and Results Act (GPRA) to report on the outcomes being achieved by their program. Despite this requirement, no data on outcomes for two federal programs serving young children with disabilities, Part C (early intervention for birth to 2-year-olds) and Part B Preschool Grants Program (early childhood special education for 3- to 5-year-olds) of IDEA were reported for many years. No data collection mechanism was in place that could regularly produce data on child outcomes, nor was it clear how such data collection could ever be implemented given the numerous challenges associated with assessing a population that was very young and extremely hetero-geneous in development (National Research Council, 2008). To better align spending with demonstrated program effectiveness, the federal Office of Management and Budget instituted a new review process in 2002 that involved giving scores to programs based on the kinds of data the program had available. Both the Part C and the Part B Pre-school Grants Program received a score of zero for results and accountability and a summative assessment of "Results Not Demon-strated." Given that the rationale for the review was to guide future budgeting decisions, the outcome of this review led the federal agency responsible for overseeing these two programs to immediately under-take action to obtain data on child outcomes. The federal government required that each state provide data on progress toward three child outcomes (social relationships, acquisition of knowledge and skills, and the taking of appropriate action to take needs) for all children receiving services through EI or ECSE programs. States submitted data to address this requirement for the first time in 2007. As states build their measurement systems, they have been able to report data on a higher percentage of children participating in these two programs with each subsequent year. More detailed information about the data requirements and state approaches to the data collection can be found in Hebbeler, Barton, and Mallik (2008) and Hebbeler and Rooney (2009), and at –http://www.the–ECO-Center.org.

Once state measurement systems are fully developed, data on out-comes for young children with disabilities will be available for over one million children nationally. These data will be available for each state and for local programs within states. Since some state databases also include data on cost of services, calculating the cost-effectiveness of services for children in a variety of programs in some states could be a relatively straightforward analysis. The availability of good data on child outcomes will allow programs to carry out the requirement of IDEA 2004 for states to monitor on child outcomes. The child outcomes data has the potential to help identify weak areas in the state system of services; the data could pinpoint less effective programs or weak components of the statewide system such as insufficient support for promoting children's independence through assistive technology. It also has the potential to be misused in some of the same ways that accountability data has been misused in K–12 education, which is why states and programs have been cautioned on appropriate interpretation and use (Early Childhood Outcomes Center, 2004) The burgeoning capacity of states to reach conclusions about cost-effectiveness is not imminent and depends on the quality of the outcomes data and the availability of cost data in the states. A recent survey of states found that only 20 of the 38 states responding had data on the amount of services delivered in early intervention (IDEA Infant and Toddlers Coordinators Association, 2009), suggesting it will be many years before states routinely are able to link data on service costs to outcomes. As states build their systems for ongoing child outcomes measurement and move to better and more thorough information on services, the groundwork is being laid for the creation of much-needed information about the cost-effectiveness of services, Unlike the cost-effectiveness information of the past, which was time-limited and available only for a small set of program models or features, this will be ongoing information available from year to year for use in building more effective and efficient services delivery systems.

One other emerging trend with the potential to substantially increase the ongoing availability of data on outcomes is the development of longitudinal data systems in education. Supported by federal funds, nearly all states are now undertaking to build data systems that allow the state education agency to track student progress across years (Data Quality Campaign, 2008). More recently, states are moving to add information from early childhood programs to these data systems (Early Childhood Data Collaborative, 2010). A small number of states can already track children from early intervention through high school graduation. Longitudinal data systems that link EI and ECSE information to K–12 will allow states to calculate the proportion of children who no longer need special services and track their educational achievement in future years as well as address a variety of questions about the relationship between program participation in early childhood and long-term outcomes. This kind of information also will provide the necessary information for economic analyses that examine cost savings associated with early childhood services or look at the cost-effectiveness of alternate programming approaches provided before age 5.

CONCLUSIONS

The strong interest of policymakers and the general public in knowing more about the costs and outcomes of a full range of social service, health and education programs is likely to continue. As there has been for many years now, there is a pressing need to move beyond justifying budget requests for programs for children with disabilities with anecdotal evidence and generic research on brain development or even efficacy studies of what can work. We need data on how funded programs are improving outcomes and what kinds of approaches are cost-effective. Although we would want to believe that all components of the service delivery system are working in a highly effective manner for all children and families being served, it is not likely to be the case. And if it is not the case, then the only way to address this situation is with better information to pinpoint and address weaknesses. Both families and taxpayers are entitled to services that are cost-effective.

This overview of what is known about costs, efficacy, and cost-effectiveness of programs for young children with disability reveals a persistent need for new and better information. Although there are several challenges to conducting good studies in this area, that is no reason not to make progress in this area. The need for the information is not lessened by challenges such as the diversity of the population, mandated individualized services, and the variety of service delivery approaches. We have tried to elucidate the distinctions between the knowledge of what works that is acquired in controlled settings, which constitutes our research literature on efficacy, and the knowledge of how these practices are implemented in programs across the country. We need to continue to do more research to validate new promising practices and identify the children and families with whom they are successful. We also need to do much more to learn about what can work, what is being implemented, and what is working in the hundreds of early intervention and early childhood special education programs across the country. We need ongoing data on the outcomes children are realizing through their participation in these programs. Collecting this information will not involve random assignment to conditions, nor should it, because we need information on the outcomes being realized in programs as they operate day to day. The efficacy literature demonstrates that programs *can be* effective. The current need is for ongoing data to identify which programs are and are not effective. Information on child outcomes is needed at many levels to support good decision making by teachers and other practitioners, administrators, and policy makers.

Cost of programs, services, and practices is another area about which we currently know very little. For cost data to be usable and useful, it needs to be current, which means it needs to be produced regularly. Cost data on programs from 5 or 10 years ago might be useful for a onetime exploration of what is driving costs, but we would argue that both outcomes and cost data need to be tracked from year to year. The cost-effectiveness data that results from combining these two pieces of information may be a long way off, but represent the strongest kind of information for effective program management. Currently, we have no way of knowing which of our EI and ECSE dollars are good investments and which are not. There are far too few resources and far too many families who need quality services and supports for this to be acceptable.

Calling for cost-effectiveness to strengthen our investments in programs for young children is not the same as calling for a cost-benefit analysis to justify those investments. Barnett and Escobar (2002) commented that the time had come for analysis of programs for children with environmental risks to move from showing that programs are economically efficient to looking at how programs can produce the greatest benefit at the lowest cost. Similarly, the question for services for children with disabilities should not be whether the short- and long-term outcomes justify the investment (although the data would indicate that the answer to this question is yes). The critical cost question for programs for young children with disabilities is, how do we provide effective services for the greatest number of children at the least cost? This should not be misconstrued as a justification for automatically providing the least expensive services because a low-cost (or high-cost) service that does not result in a good outcome is not cost-effective. Examining cost-effectiveness means looks at the amount of gain achieved for a given level of investment, which is what decision makers need to know to make choices among options. Obtaining valid data on cost-effectiveness will not be easy, but if we do not start investing soon to build the infrastructure in states to collect it, another 25 years will go by and the field will still be writing about the need for data on cost-effectiveness.

The European Academy of Child Disability presents an interesting position on the effectiveness of services: "Health providers have a responsibility to try to measure the effectiveness of any programs set up for children with disabilities and to identify which treatments are ineffective. On the other hand the availability of certain services such as early intervention is now an accepted right, even though appropriate evaluation methods may be lacking" (McConachie, Smyth, & Bax, 1997; Blackman, 2000, p. 14). We know enough to know that programs for young children with disabilities can make a substantial difference in their lives, and for that reason alone, these programs need to be funded. Now we need to learn enough to ensure that every program and service lives up to that potential.

REFERENCES

American Academy of Pediatrics Committee on Children with Disabilities. (2001). Developmental surveillance and screening of infants and young children. *Pediatrics, 108*, 192–196.

Anderson, L. M., Shinn, C., Fullilove, M. T., Scrimshaw, S. C., Fielding, J. E., Normand, J., et al. (2003). The effectiveness of early childhood development programs: A systematic review. *American Journal of Preventive Medicine, 24*(3S), 32–46.

Bailey, D. B., Jr., Bruder, M. B., Hebbeler, K., Carta, J., deFosset, M., Greenwood, C., et al. (2006). Recommended outcomes for families of young children with disabilities. *Journal of Early Intervention, 28*(4), 227–251.

Barnett, S. W., & Hustedt, J. T. (2005). Head Start's lasting benefits. *Infants & Young Children, 18*(1), 16–24.

Barnett, W. S. (2000). Economics of early childhood intervention. In J. P. Shonkoff & S. J. Meisels (Eds.), *Handbook of early childhood intervention* (2nd ed., pp. 589–612). New York: Cambridge University Press.

Barnett, W. S., & Escobar, C. M. (1988). The economics of early intervention for handicapped children: What do we really know? *Journal of Early Intervention, 12*(2), 169–181.

Barnett, W. S., & Escobar, C. M. (2002). Research on the cost effectiveness of early educational intervention: Implications for research and policy. *American Journal of Community Psychology, 17*(6), 677–704.

Barnett, W. S., & Masse, L. N. (2007). Comparative benefit-cost analysis of the Abecedarian program and its policy implications. *Economics of Education Review, 26*(1), 113–125.

Belfield, C., Nores, M., Barnett, W. S., & Schweinhart, L. J. (2006). The High/Scope Perry Preschool Program: Cost-benefit analysis using data from the age-40 followup. *Journal of Human Resources, 41*(1), 162–190.

Blackman, J. A. (2000). Early intervention: A global perspective. *Infants and Young Children, 15*(2), 11–19.

Bricker, D. (2000). Inclusion: How the scene has changed. *Topics in Early Childhood Special Education, 20*(1), 14–19.

Buysse, V., & Bailey, D. B. (1993). Behavioral and developmental outcomes in young children with disabilities in integrated and segregated settings: A review of comparative studies. *Journal of Special Education, 26*, 434–461.

Chambers, J. (1991, Fall). A cost analysis of the federal program for early intervention services. *Journal of Education Finance, 17*, 142–171.

Chambers, J. G., & Parrish, T. B. (1994). Modeling resource costs. In S. Barnett & H. Walberg (Eds.), *Cost analysis for educational decision making.* Greenwich, CT: JAI Press.

Chasson, G., Harris, G., & Neely, W. (2007). Cost comparison of early intensive behavioral intervention and special education for children with autism. *Journal of Child and Family Studies, 16*(3), 401–413.

Cooper, J. O., Heron, T. E., & Heward, W. L. (2007). *Applied behavior analysis* (2nd ed.). Prentice Hall.

Cunningham, C. C., Bremner, R., & Boyle, M. (1995). Large group community-based parenting programs for families of preschoolers at risk for disruptive behavioral disorders: Utilization, sot effectiveness, and outcomes. *Journal of Child Psychology and Psychiatry, 36*, 1141–1159.

Currie, J., & Thomas, D. (1995). Does Head Start make a difference? *American Economic Review, 85*(3), 341–364.

Data Quality Campaign. (2008). Measuring what matters: Creating longitudinal data systems to improve student achievement Retrieved from http://www.dataqualitycampaign.org/files/DQC_measuring_what_matter

DEC/NAEYC. (2009). Early childhood inclusion: A summary. Chapel Hill: University of North Carolina, FPG Child Development Institute.

Dobrez, D., Sasso, A. L., Holl, J., Shalowitz, M., Leon, S., & Budetti, P. (2001). Estimating the cost of developmental and behavioral screening of school children in general pediatric practice. *Pediatrics, 108*, 913–922.

Dunst, C. J., Trivette, C. M., & Jodry, W. (1997). Influences of social support on children with disabilities and their families. In M. J. Guralnick (Ed.), *The effectiveness of early intervention*. Baltimore: Paul H. Brookes Publishing.

Early Childhood Data Collaborative. (2010). Building and using coordinated state early care and education data systems: A framework for state policy makers. Retrieved from http://www.dataqualitycampaign.org/files/DQC%20ECDC%20WhitePaper%20FINAL%20online.pdf

Early Childhood Outcomes Center. (2004). Uses and misuses of data on outcomes for children with disabilities. Retrieved from http://www.the-eco-center.org

Eiserman, W. D., McCoun, M., & Escobar, C. M. (1996). A cost-effectiveness analysis of two alternative program models for serving speech-disordered preschoolers. *British Medical Journal, 312*, 1655–1658.

Erickson, M. (1992). An analysis of early intervention expenditures in Massachusetts. *American Journal on Mental Retardation, 96*(6), 617–629.

Escobar, C. M., Barnett, W. S., & Goetze, L. D. (1994). Cost analysis in early intervention. *Journal of Early Intervention, 18*(1), 48–63.

Farran, D. C. (1990). Effects of intervention with disadvantages and disabled children: A decade review. In J. P. Shonkoff & S. J. Meisels (Eds.), *Handbook of early intervention* (2nd ed., pp. 201–539). Cambridge: Cambridge University Press.

Farran, D. C. (2000). Another decade of intervention for children who are low income or disabled: What do we know now? In J. P. Shonkoff & S. J. Meisels (Eds.), *Handbook of early childhood intervention* (2nd ed., pp. 510–548). New York: Cambridge University Press.

Fuchs, D., & Fuchs, L. (1994). Inclusive schools movement and the radicalization of special education reform. *Exceptional Children, 60*, 294–309.

Gallagher, J. J., Clayton, J. R., & Heinemeier, S. E. (2001). Education for four-year-olds: State initiatives. Chapel Hill: University of North Carolina.

Gardner, W. I. (2006). *Behavior modification in mental retardation*. New York: Aldine De Gruyter.

Gibson, D., & Harris, A. (1988). Aggregated early intervention effects for Down's syndrome persons: Patterning and longevity of benefits. *Journal of Mental Deficiency Research, 32*, 1–17.

Glascoe, F. P., Foster, E. M., & Wolraich, M. L. (1997). An economic analysis of developmental detection methods. *Pediatrics, 99*(6), 830–837.

Guralnick, M. J. (1989). Recent developments in early intervention efficacy research: Implications for family involvement in P.L. 99-457. *Topics in Early Childhood Special Education, 9,* 1–17.

Guralnick, M. J. (2001). Connections between developmental science and intervention science. *Zero to Three: The Science of Early Childhood Development, 21,* 24–29.

Guralnick, M. J. (2005a). Inclusion as a core principle in the early intervention system. In M. J. Guralnick (Ed.), *The developmental systems approach to early intervention* (pp. 59–69). Baltimore: Paul H. Brookes Publishing.

Guralnick, M. J. (Ed.). (1997). *The effectiveness of early intervention.* Baltimore: Paul H. Brookes Publishing.

Guralnick, M. J. (Ed.). (2001). *Early childhood inclusion.* Baltimore: Paul H. Brookes Publishing.

Guralnick, M. J. (Ed.). (2005b). *The developmental systems approach to early intervention.* Baltimore: Paul H. Brookes Publishing.

Guralnick, M. J., & Bricker, D. (1987). The effectiveness of early intervention for children with cognitive and general developmental delays. In M. J. Guralnick & F. C. Bennett (Eds.), *The effectiveness of early intervention for at-risk and handicapped children* (pp. 115–173). New York: Academic Press.

Guralnick, M. J., Neville, B., Hammond, M. A., & Connor, R. T. (2008). Continuity and change from full-inclusion early childhood programs through the early elementary period. *Journal of Early Intervention, 30*(3), 237–250.

Hart, B., & Risley, T. (1995). *Meaningful differences in the everyday experience of young American children.* Baltimore: Paul H. Brookes Publishing.

Hatch, O. G. (1984). Environmental constraints affecting services for the handicapped. *Topics in Early Childhood Special Education, 4*(1), 83–90.

Hebbeler, K., Barton, L., & Mallik, S. (2008). Assessment and accountability for programs serving young children with disabilities. *Exceptionality*(16), 48–63.

Hebbeler, K., Levin, J., Perez, M., Lam, I., & Chambers, J. (2009). Expenditures for early intervention services. *Infants and Young Children, 22*(2), 76–86.

Hebbeler, K., & Rooney, R. (2009, October). Accountability for services for young children with disabilities and the assessment of meaningful outcomes: The role of the speech-language pathologist. *Language, Speech, and Hearing Services in Schools, 40,* 446–456

Hebbeler, K., Spiker, D., Morrison, K., & Mallik, S. (2008). A national look at the characteristics of Part C early intervention services. *Young Exceptional Children Monograph Series No. 10.*

Heckman, J. J., & Masterov, D. V. (2004). The productivity argument for investing in young children. Washington, DC: Invest in Kids Working Group, Committee for Economic Development.

Hemmeter, M. L. (2000). Classroom-based interventions: Evaluating the past and looking toward the future. *Topics in Early Childhood Special Education, 20*(1), 56–61.

Hogan, C. (2001). The power of outcomes: Strategic thinking to improve results for our children, families, and communities (p. 13). Washington, DC: National Governors Association.

Howes, C., Burchinal, M., Pianta, R., Bryant, D., Early, D., Clifford, R., et al. (2008). Ready to learn? Children's pre-academic achievement in pre-kindergarten programs? *Early Childhood Research Quarterly, 23*(2), 27–50.

Hummel-Rossi, B., & Ashdown, J. (2002). The state of cost-benefit and cost-effectiveness analyses in education. *Review of Educational Research, 72*(1), 1–30. doi: 10.3102/00346543072001001

IDEA Infant and Toddlers Coordinators Association. (2009). Part C Implementation: State challenges and responses Retrieved from http://www.ideainfanttoddler.org/pdf/09_Annual_Survey_Report-State_Challenges.pdf

Jacobson, J. W., Mulick, J. A., & Green, G. (1998). Cost-benefit estimates for early intensive behavioral intervention for young children with autism—general model and single state case. *Behavioral Interventions, 13*, 201–226.

Karen, R., Helfand, M., Homer, C., McPhillips, H., & Lieu, T. A. (2002). Projected cost-effectiveness of statewide universal newborn hearing screening. *Pediatrics, 110*, 855–864.

Karoly, L. A. (2005). County-level estimates of the effects of a universal preschool program in California. Santa Monica, CA: RAND Corporation.

Karoly, L. A., & Bigelow, J. H. (2005). The economics of investing in universal preschool education in California (p. 235). Santa Monica, CA: RAND Corporation.

Karoly, L. A., Greenwood, P. W., Everingham, S. S., Hoube, J., Kilburn, M. R., Rydell, C. P., et al. (1998). Investing in our children: What we know and don't know about the costs and benefits of early childhood interventions. Santa Monica, CA: RAND Corporation.

Karoly, L. A., Kilburn, M. R., Bigelow, J. H., Caulkins, J. P., & Cannon, J. (2001). Assessing costs and benefits of early childhood intervention programs: Overview and application to the Starting Early Starting Smart Program. Santa Monica, CA: RAND Corporation.

Karoly, L. A., Kilburn, M. R., & Cannon, J. S. (2005). Early childhood interventions: Proven results, future promise. Santa Monica, CA: RAND Corporation.

Kauerz, K. (2001). Starting early starting now: A policymaker's guide to early care and education and school success (pp. 27). Denver, CO: Education Commission of the States.

Kelly, J. F., Booth-LaForce, C., & Spieker, S. J. (2005). Assessing family characteristics relevant to early intervention. In M. J. Guralnick (Ed.), *The developmental systems approach to early intervention* (pp. 235–265). Baltimore: Paul H. Brookes Publishing.

Koegel, R. L., & Koegel, L. K. (2006). *Pivotal response treatments for autism.* Baltimore: Paul H. Brookes Publishing.

Lee, V. E., & Burkam, D. T. (2002). Inequality at the starting gate: Social background differences in achievement as children begin school. Washington, DC: Economic Policy Institute.

Levin, H. M. (1983). *Cost-effectiveness: A primer.* Beverly HIlls, CA: SAGE Publications.

Levin, H. M., & McEwan, P. J. (2000). *Cost effectivenss analysis: Methods and applications.* Thousand Oaks, CA: SAGE Publications.

Levin, J., Perez, M., Lam, I., Chambers, J. G., & Hebbeler, K. M. (2004). National Early Intervention Longitudinal Study: Expenditure Study. Menlo Park, CA: SRI International.

Lord, C., Wagner, A., Rogers, S., Szatmari, P., Aman, M., Charman, T., et al. (2005). Challenges in evaluating psychosocial interventions for autistic spectrum disorders. *Journal of Autism and Developmental Disorders, 35*(6), 695–708.

Lovaas, O. I. (1987). Behavioral treatment and normal intellectual and educational functioning in autistic children. *Journal of Consulting and Clinical Psychology, 55*, 3–9.

Mackey-Andrews, S. D., & Taylor, A. (2007). *To fee or not to fee: That is the question!* (NECTAC Notes, No. 22) Chapel Hill: University of North Carolina, FPG Child Development Institute, National Early Childhood Technical Assistance Center.

Macy, D. J., & Schafer, D. S. (1985). Real-time cost analysis: Application in early intervention. *Journal of Early Intervention, 9*(2), 98–104.

Mahoney, G., Boyce, G., Fewell, R. R., Spiker, D., & Wheeden, C. A. (1998). The relationship of parent-child interaction to the effectiveness of early intervention services for at-risk children and children with disabilities. *Topics in Early Childhood Special Education, 18*, 5–17.

Mahoney, G., & Perales, F. (2005). Relationship-focused intervention with children with pervasive developmental disorders and other disabilities: A comparative study. *Journal of Developmental and Behavioral Pediatrics, 26*, 77–85.

McCathren, R. B., Yoder, P. J., & Warren, S. F. (1995). The role of directives in early language intervention. *Journal of Early Intervention, 19*, 91–101.

McConachie, H., Smyth, D., & Bax, M. (1997). Services for children with disabilities in European countries. *Developmental Medicine and Child Neurology, 39*, 5.

Mehl, A. L., & Thomson, V. (1998). Newborn Hearing Screening: The Great Omission. *Pediatrics, 101*(1), e4.

Morley, E., Vinson, E., & Hatry, H. P. (2000). A look at outcome measurement in nonprofit agencies. Washington, DC: Urban Institute.

Murray, C. J. L., Evans, D. B., Acharya, A., & Baltussen, R. M. P. M. (2000). Development of WHO guidelines in generalized cost-effectiveness analysis. *Health Economics, 9*(3), 235–251. doi: 10.1002/(SICI)1099-1050(200004)9:3<235::AID-HEC502>3.0.CO;2-O

National Governors Association. (2005). Building the foundation for bright futures: Final report of the NGA Task Force on School Readiness. Washington, DC: National Governors Association.

National Research Council. (2008). Early childhood assessment: Why, what, and how? Committee on Developmental Outcomes and Assessments for Young Children, Catherine E. Snow and Susan B. Van Hemel,(Eds.). Board on Children, Youth and Families, Board on Testing and Assessment, Division of Behavioral and Social Sciences and Education. Washington, DC: The National Academies.

National Research Council and Institute of Medicine. (2000). *From neurons to neighborhoods: The science of early childhood development.* Washington, DC: National Academy Press.

National Research Council and Institute of Medicine. (2009). Strengthening benefit-cost analysis for early childhood interventions: Workshop summary *A. Beatty, Rapporteur. Committee on Strengthening Benefit-Cost Methodology for the Evaluation of Early Childhood Interventions, Board on Children, Youth, and Families. Division of Behavioral and Social Sciences and Education.* Washington, DC: National Academies Press.

Odom, S. L., Hanson, M. J., Lieber, J., Marquart, J., Sandall, S., Wolery, R., et al. (2001). The costs of preschool inclusion. *Topics in Early Childhood Special Education, 21*(1), 46–55.

President's Commission on Excellence in Special Education. (2002). A new era: Revitalizing special education for children and their families. Washington, DC: U.S. Department of Education.

Reynolds, A. J., Temple, J. A., Robertson, D. L., & Mann, E. A. (2002). Age 21 cost-benefit analysis of the Title I Chicago Child-Parent Centers. *Educational Evaluation and Policy Analysis, 24*(4), 267–303.

Roberts, R. N., Innocenti, M. S., & Goetze, L. D. (1999). Emerging issues from state level evaluations of early intervention programs. *Journal of Early Intervention, 22* (2), 152–163.

Roper, N., & Dunst, C. J. (2003). Communication interventions in natural environments: Guidelines for practice. *Infants and Young Children, 16,* 215–226.

Scarborough, A., Spiker, D., Mallik, S., Hebbeler, K. M., Bailey, D., & Simeonsson, R. (2004). A national look at children and families entering early intervention. *Exceptional Children, 70,* 469–483.

Scarborough, A. A., Hebbeler, K. M., & Spiker, D. (2006). Eligibility characteristics of infants and toddlers entering early intervention in the United States. *Journal of Policy and Practice in Intellectual Disabilities, 3*(1), 57–64.

Schweinhart, L. J. (2004). The High/Scope Perry Preschool Study through age 40: Summary, conclusions, and frequently asked questions. Ypsilanti, MI: High/Scope Educational Research Foundation.

Schweinhart, L. J., Montie, J., Xiang, Z., Barnett, W. S., Belfield, C. R., & Nores, M. (2005). Lifetime effects: The High/Scope Perry Preschool Study through age 40 (p. 18). Ypsilanti, MI: High/Scope Press.

Shonkoff, J. P., & Meisels, S. J. (Eds.). (2000). *Handbook of early childhood intervention* (2nd ed.). New York: Cambridge University Press.

Spiker, D., Boyce, G., & Boyce, L. (2002). Parent-child interactions when infants and young children have disabilities. In L. Gidden (Ed.), *International Review of Research in Mental Retardation* (Vol. 25, pp. 35–70). San Diego, CA: Academic Press.

Spiker, D., & Hebbeler, K. (1999). Early intervention services. In M. Levine, W. B. Carey, & A. C. Crocker (Eds.), *Developmental-Behavioral Pediatrics* (3rd ed., pp. 793–802). Philadelphia, PA: W. B. Saunders Company.

Spiker, D., Hebbeler, K., & Mallik, S. (2005). Developing and implementing early intervention programs for children with established disabilities. In M. J. Guralnick (Ed.), *The developmental systems approach to early intervention* (pp. 305–349). Baltimore: Paul H. Brookes Publishing.

Spiker, D., & Hopmann, M. R. (1997). The effectiveness of early intervention for children with Down Syndrome. In M. J. Guralnick (Ed.), *The effectiveness of early intervention* (pp. 271–306). Baltimore: Paul H. Brookes Publishing.

Squires, J., Nickels, R. E., & Eisart, D. (1996). Early Detection of Developmental Problems: Strategies for Monitoring Young Children in the Practice Setting. *Journal of Developmental and Behavioral Pediatrics, 17,* 420–427.

Tarr, J. E., & Barnett, W. S. (2001). A cost analysis of Part C early intervention services in new jersey. *Journal of Early Intervention, 24*(1), 45–54. doi: 10.1177/105381510102400107

Taylor, C., White, K. R., & Pezzino, J. (1984). Cost-effectiveness analysis of full-day versus half-day intervention programs for handicapped preschoolers. *Journal of Early Intervention, 9,* 76–85.

Taylor, M. J., White, K. R., & Kusmierek, A. (1993). The cost-effectiveness of increasing hours per week of early intervention services for young children with disabilities. *Early Education and Development, 4*(4), 238–255.

Temple, J. A., & Reynolds, A. J. (2007). Benefits and costs of investments in preschool education: Evidence from the Child-Parent Centers and related programs. *Economics of Education Review, 26,* 126–144.

Wagner, M., Blackorby, J., Cameto, R., Hebbeler, K., & Newman, L. (1993). The transition experiences of young people with disabilities: A summary of findings from NLTS. Menlo Park, CA: SRI International.

Warfield, M. E. (1994). A cost-effectiveness analysis of early intervention services in Massachusetts: Implications for policy. *Educational Evaluation and Policy Analysis, 16*(1), 87–99. doi: 10.3102/01623737016001087

Warren, S. F. (2000). The future of early communication and language intervention. *Topics in Early Childhood Special Education, 20,* 33–37.

Webster-Stratton, C. (1997). Early intervention for families of preschool children with conduct problems. In M. J. Guralnick (Ed.), *The effectiveness of early intervention.* Baltimore: Paul H. Brookes Publishing.

Wolery, M. (2000). Behavioral and educational approaches to early intervention. In J. P. Shonkoff & S. J. Meisels (Eds.), *Handbook of early childhood intervention* (2nd ed., pp. 179–203). New York: Cambridge University Press.

Wolery, M., & Wilbers, J. S. (Eds.). (1994). *Including children with special needs in early childhood programs.* Washington, DC: National Association for the Education of Young Children.

Yoder, P. J., & Warren, S. F. (2004). Early predictors of language in children with and without Down syndrome. *American Journal of Mental Retardation, 109,* 285–300.

Yoshinaga-Itano, C. (2004). Levels of evidence: Universal newborn hearing screening (UNHS) and early hearing detection and intervention systems (EHDI). *Journal of Communication Disorders, 37,* 451–465.

Zill, N., Resnick, G., Kim, K., O'Donnell, K., Sorongon, A., McKey, R. H., et al. (2003). Head Start FACES 2000: A whole-child perspective on program performance (fourth progress report). Washington, DC: U.S. Department of Health and Human Services.

About the Editor and Contributors

EDITOR

Steven Eidelman, MBA, MSW, is the University of Delaware's H. Rodney Sharp Professor of Human Services Policy and Leadership. Mr. Eidelman also has an academic appointment as the University of Delaware's first Robert Edelsohn Chair in Disabilities Studies. He holds joint faculty appointments in the School of Urban Affairs and Public Policy and the Department of Individual and Family Studies. He has served as executive director of both the Association for Retarded Citizens of the United States and the Joseph P. Kennedy Jr. Foundation. Mr. Eidelman is well known for his support to families and individuals with disabilities and for his broad national and international network in the field of disabilities.

CONTRIBUTORS

Lizanne DeStefano, PhD, is Professor in Quantitative and Evaluative Research Methodologies in Educational Psychology at the University of Illinois, Urbana-Champaign. She has done research on the evaluations of initiatives such as NCLB, Head Start, the National Assessment of Educational Progress, Part H of IDEA, the transition requirements of IDEA, Goals 2000 legislation, and the National Youth Sports Program. She uses both qualitative and quantitative research methods to evaluate the impact of policies in a local scale. Dr. DeStefano is currently director of the I-STEM Education Initiative at the University of Illinois to promote students' interest and performance in science, technology, engineering, and mathematics.

Joan C. Eichner, MPA, MPH, is the Children's Policy Director at the University of Pittsburgh Office of Child Development (OCD). She has been involved with maternal and child health, mental health services, homeless and housing services, and international development in the public and nonprofit sectors. In her current position, Ms. Eichner supports the work of the Policy Initiatives Division at OCD, which seeks to change policy and practice to improve outcomes for children and families by informing policy makers of relevant research, best practices, and evaluation results. She currently works on a range of projects in early childhood, including mental health, early intervention, young children experiencing homelessness, and strategic planning and communications. These duties combine her training in public health and public administration with her dedication to working in partnership with families and communities.

Susan A. Fowler, PhD, is Professor in Special Education at the University of Illinois Urbana-Champaign. Her research interests are the development of intervention strategies to enhance young children's language, social, and cognitive development and the development of guidelines and practices to help communities and programs coordinate delivery of services to children and families. Dr. Fowler has coauthored and implemented curriculums such as "Spark!" for the development of early literacy.

Christina Groark, PhD, is a mother of three children, one of whom has special needs. Her MEd and PhD are in education for young children. She is Co-Director of the University of Pittsburgh Office of Child Development and Associate Professor in the School of Education at the University of Pittsburgh. Her major areas of scholarly expertise include the design, implementation, and management of collaborative service intervention for infants and young children, children with disabilities; and practice and policy pertaining to at-risk children and families. She is known internationally for her work with institutions for children without permanent parental care. Dr. Groark is coauthor of *The Effects of Early Social-Emotional and Relationship Experience on the Development of Young Orphanage Children* (2008), a Monograph of the Society for Research in Child Development, and is primary editor of *Evidence-Based Practices and Programs for Early Childhood Care and Education* (2007). She has also written extensively on early care and education, the integration of developmental scholarship into practice and policy, and university-community collaborations. Her research in interventions to improve the lives of institutionalized children and the Long-Term Effects of Early Social-Emotional Experience is funded by NIMH and by private sponsors like Half the Sky Foundation and Whole Child International. Her research has been developed in orphanages in Latin America, Russia, and recently in China. Dr. Groark is the recipient of the University of Pittsburgh's 2005 Chancellor's Award for Public Service and the University of Pittsburgh School of Education's 2009 Faculty Research Award.

Kathleen Hebbeler is part of the Early Childhood Outcomes (ECO) Center. The ECO Center is a collaborative effort of SRI (Stanford Research Institute) International, the University of North Carolina's Frank Porter Graham Child Development Institute, RTI International, and the University of Connecticut. ECO provides national leadership in assisting states with the implementation of high-quality outcome systems for early intervention and early childhood special education programs.

Susan P. Maude, PhD, is an Associate Professor in the Department of Human Development and Family Studies, College of Human Sciences at Iowa State University. Her research interests include inclusive personnel preparation, program evaluation in early intervention and early childhood special education, and innovative ways to evaluate diversity within programs. She is past-president of the Division for Early Childhood (DEC) at the Council for Exceptional Children. DEC is a national organization dedicated to promoting policies and practices that aid the development of young children with special needs.

Michaelene M. Ostrosky, PhD, focuses much of her research on the social and emotional development of young children with special needs. Her research interests focus on (1) facilitating positive attitudes of kindergarteners toward their peers with disabilities, (2) promoting the social and communicative behavior of young children with disabilities, and (3) preparing personnel in early childhood special education.

Oleg Palmov, PhD, is Director of Infant Clinical Psychology Training and Associate Professor at the Department of Social Adjustment and Psychosocial Support in the Faculty of Psychology at St. Petersburg State University (Russian Federation). His primary research interests are infant mental health, children with disabilities, and interventions for infants and young children.

Beth Rous, PhD, is Professor of Educational Leadership Studies at the University of Kentucky. She is coauthor with Barbara Smith of a seminal chapter called *Policy in Early Childhood Education and Early Intervention: What Every Early Childhood Educator Needs to Know*. Dr. Rouss has worked on topics such as preschool accountability systems, transition to public preschool for young children with disabilities, and family stress and resources. She is part of the Human Development Institute at the University of Kentucky, a center for excellence in developmental disabilities education, research, and service.

Bruce K. Shapiro, MD, is Professor of Pediatrics at the Johns Hopkins University School of Medicine and the Arnold J. Capute, MD, MPH Chair in Neurodevelopmental Disabilities. He is Vice President of Training and Associate Director of the Maternal and Child Health Training Program, "Leadership Education Excellence in Caring for Children with Neurodevelopmental and related Disabilities" (LEND). He is also Director of the Kennedy Krieger Institute/Johns Hopkins University Neurodevelopmental Disabilities Residency Program. His research focuses on identification, assessment, and therapy of neuro-development disorders.

Barbara J. Smith, PhD, is Research Professor at the School of Education and Human Development University of Colorado, Denver. Dr. Smith has served as Executive Director of the Division for Early Childhood (DEC) of the Council for Exceptional Children (CEC). She has also served as Assistant Executive Director at the Early Learning Institute in Pittsburgh, Pennsylvania. Dr. Smith has wide experience in early childhood education programs, career development and service delivery for children. Dr. Smith is coauthor of the *DEC Recommended Practices in Early Intervention/Early Childhood Special Education* (2000). She has received several grants for research in socio-emotional interventions, special education and foundations of early learning.

Donna Spiker, PhD, is Program Manager of the Early Childhood Program at SRI (Stanford Research Institute) International. Dr. Spiker is a developmental psychologist with extensive experience designing and conducting research and evaluations on the effects of early intervention, early care and education, and school readiness programs for infants and young children with disabilities and their families. Dr. Spiker is principal investigator of the evaluation of the St. Paul Early Childhood Scholarship Pilot Program, the Pre-Kindergarten

Allowances Project for the Minnesota Early Learning Foundation, and the Illinois Early Childhood Block Grant Program for the Illinois State Board of Education. She previously codirected the Statewide Data Collection and Evaluation of First 5 California Funded Programs, focusing on evaluation of the School Readiness Initiative and the Special Needs Project. She codirected the National Early Intervention Longitudinal Study (NEILS), the first national study of early intervention for infant and toddlers with disabilities.

Bahira Sherif Trask, PhD, is Professor in the Department of Human Development and Family Studies at the University of Delaware (UD) and holds a joint appointment at the Center for Community Development and Family Policy in UD. She is interested in the global context in which family processes unfold. Her current research is funded by the Annie E. Casey Foundation to examine the interrelationship between family, work, and gender roles as well as intergenerational relationships between adult children and their parents from the perspective of family support and community economic development.

Tweety Yates, PhD, received her doctorate from the University of Illinois. Dr. Yates's research interests include parent-child interaction and personnel development issues in early childhood. Her research has focused on the validity and feasibility of a parent-child relationship-based model of early intervention in culturally and geographically diverse settings. She is also involved in training and evaluation of an early literacy staff development program with preschoolers living at or below poverty.

Advisory Board

Heidi M. Feldman, MD, PhD, is the Ballinger-Swindles Endowed Professor of Developmental and Behavioral Pediatrics at Stanford University School of Medicine. She also serves as the Medical Director of the Developmental and Behavior Pediatric Programs at Lucile Packard Children's Hospital. Dr. Feldman received her BA in Psychology (1970), summa cum laude, and her PhD in Developmental Psychology (1975) from the University of Pennsylvania. She received her MD from the University of California, San Diego (1979). Dr. Feldman has memberships in several professional societies such as the Society for Research in Child Development, the Society for Pediatric Research, and the American Academy of Pediatrics. She has served as President at the Society for the Developmental Behavioral Pediatrics. Her research focuses on developmental-behavioral pediatrics, language development in young children, and language and cognition after prematurity. She has published more than 50 peer-reviewed articles in journals like the *New England Journal of Medicine, Science, Brain and Language, Child Development, Journal of Behavioral Developmental Pediatrics, Developmental Neuropsychology,* and *Pediatrics*. She is one of the editors of the current edition of the premier textbook in her field, *Developmental-Behavioral Pediatrics* (4th ed.), published in 2009. She has served as grant reviewer for the National Institutes of Health (1992–1997 and 2008–2012) and an abstract reviewer for the Pediatric Academic Societies. Dr. Feldman has held several academic appointments: Professor at the Medical Center Line, Stanford University (2006 to present), Professor in Pediatrics, University of Pittsburgh (2000–2006), and Faculty Member at the Center for the Neural Bases of Cognition at the University of Pittsburgh/Carnegie Mellon University (2003–2006). Dr. Feldman has received several awards such as Best Doctors in America (2007–2008 and 2009–2010), Academy of Master Educators, University of Pittsburgh School of

Medicine (2006), Outstanding Alumna, University of California San Diego (2003), Ronald L. and Patricia M. Violi Professor of Pediatrics and Child Development, University of Pittsburgh (2001–2006), Excellence in Education Award, University of Pittsburgh School of Medicine (2000), and the Chancellor's Distinguished Teaching Award (1999).

Marilou Hyson, PhD, is a consultant in early child development and education and an Affiliate Faculty member in Applied Developmental Psychology at George Mason University. Formerly Associate Executive Director and Senior Consultant with the National Association for the Education of Young Children (NAEYC), Marilou contributed to the development of many position statements on issues including early learning standards, professional preparation standards, early childhood mathematics, and curriculum/assessment/program evaluation. She is the author of the recent book *Enthusiastic and Engaged Learners: Approaches to Learning in the Early Childhood Classroom*, published by NAEYC and Teachers College Press. Two book chapters on early childhood professional development and higher education systems were published in 2010. Internationally, Marilou consults in Indonesia, Bangladesh, Bhutan, and Vietnam through the World Bank and Save the Children. In the United States, Marilou consults with organizations including the Families and Work Institute, the Finance Project, the National Center for Children in Poverty, and the Society for Research in Child Development. Prior to joining NAEYC, Marilou was an SRCD Fellow in the U.S. Department of Education and Professor and Chair of the University of Delaware's Department of Individual and Family Studies. The former editor-in-chief of *Early Childhood Research Quarterly*, Marilou's research and publications have emphasized young children's emotional development, parents' and teachers' beliefs and educational practices, issues in linking research with policy and practice, and early childhood teacher preparation.

Robert Silverstein, JD, is a principal in the law firm of Powers Pyles Sutter & Verville, P.C., and he also serves as the director of the Center for the Study and Advancement of Disability Policy. Mr. Silverstein received his BS in economics, cum laude, from the Wharton School, University of Pennsylvania in 1971. He received his JD in 1974 from Georgetown University Law Center. His main areas of interest are public policy issues and the policymaking process focusing in the areas of disability, health care, rehabilitation, employment, education, social security, and civil rights. In his capacity as staff director and chief counsel to the U.S. Senate Subcommittee on Disability Policy and other positions (1986–1997), Mr. Silverstein was the behind-the-scenes architect of more than 20 bills enacted into law, including the Americans with Disabilities Act (ADA), Rehabilitation Act (1992 Amendments), the Early Intervention Program for Infants and Toddlers with Disabilities (1986), and the Individuals with Disabilities Education Act Amendments (1991, 1997 Amendments). He has presented keynotes speeches before national and state organizations and trained leaders and others in more than 40 states regarding various public policy issues and the police making process. He has more than 75 papers, articles and policy briefs on public policy issues from a disability perspective published in journals such as *Behavioral Sciences and the Law, and Iowa Law Review.* Mr. Silverstein has assisted federal, state, and local policymakers and key stakeholder groups to translate research into consensus public policy solutions addressing identified needs.

Sue Swenson is an experienced nonprofit and government leader in the field of advocacy and support for people with developmental disabilities and their families. She is interested in the application of modern management and marketing techniques to help public systems better know and serve the people they are intended to help, with a special interest in interdisciplinary applications and international collaborative efforts. Mrs. Swenson is a frequent public speaker and enthusiastic participant in forums designed to improve the lives of citizens with disabilities. She worked for The Arc of the United States as CEO. She also served as Executive Director of Joseph P. Kennedy, Jr., Foundation. She was appointed by the Clinton White House to serve as Commissioner of the Administration on Developmental Disabilities, U.S. DHHS, and served as a Kennedy Public Policy Fellow at the U.S. Senate Subcommittee on Disability Policy. Mrs. Swenson received her AB in humanities in 1975, and an AM in humanities (1977) from the University of Chicago and an MBA from the Carlson School of Management at the University of Minnesota (1986). She has three adult sons, one of whom has developmental disabilities.

Jane E. West, PhD, currently serves as Senior Vice President for Policy, Programs, and Professional Issues at the American Association of

Colleges for Teacher Education (AACTE). West has written broadly on special education, disability policy and teacher preparation. She served as the staff director for the U.S. Senate Subcommittee on Disability Policy in the early 1980s under the chairmanship of Sen. Lowell P. Weicker. She currently leads AACTE's engagement in the education policy discussion related to teacher preparation, the Elementary and Secondary Education Act and the Higher Education Act.

Index

CPSIA information can be obtained at www.ICGtesting.com
Printed in the USA
BVOW011639070213

312625BV00003B/59/P